THE SHIFT

THE SHIFT

One Nurse, Twelve Hours,
Four Patients' Lives

THERESA BROWN

ALGONQUIN BOOKS OF CHAPEL HILL   2015

Published by
Algonquin Books of Chapel Hill
Post Office Box 2225
Chapel Hill, North Carolina 27515-2225

a division of
Workman Publishing
225 Varick Street
New York, New York 10014

Published simultaneously in Canada by Thomas Allen & Son Limited.
Design by Steve Godwin.

Library of Congress Cataloging-in-Publication Data
    Brown, Theresa, author.
    The shift : one nurse, twelve hours, four patients' lives /
    Theresa Brown.—First edition.
        p. ; cm.
    ISBN 978-1-61620-320-7
    I. Title.
    [DNLM: 1. Critical Care Nursing—Pennsylvania—Personal
    Narratives. 2. Critical Care Nursing—Pennsylvania—Popular
    Works. 3. Nursing Staff, Hospital—Pennsylvania—Personal
    Narratives. 4. Nursing Staff, Hospital—Pennsylvania—Popular
    Works. 5. Intensive Care Units—Pennsylvania—Personal Narra-
    tives. 6. Intensive Care Units—Pennsylvania—Popular Works.
    7. Interprofessional Relations—Pennsylvania—Personal Narra-
    tives. 8. Interprofessional Relations—Pennsylvania—Popular
    Works. 9. Nurse-Patient Relations—Pennsylvania—Personal
    Narratives. 10. Nurse-Patient Relations—Pennsylvania—
    Popular Works. WY 154]
    RT120.I5
    616.02'8—dc23   2015010992

10 9 8 7 6 5 4 3 2 1
First Edition

To Sophia, Miranda, and Conrad—
the beginning of this journey

If all is supposition, if ending is air, then
why not happiness? Are we so cynical,
so sophisticated as to write off even the
chance of happy endings?

—TIM O'BRIEN
In the Lake of the Woods

So we come down from stony haunts—
the hypothetical eternal—to find another
way into the garden . . .
this time we'll pick the other Tree
and eat the fruit of life.

—ELEANOR WILNER
"Sarah's Choice"

Disclaimer: This book is a work of nonfiction and the stories told here are true, drawn from my time spent working as a bedside nurse on a bone-marrow transplant/medical oncology floor in a teaching hospital in Pennsylvania. Specific details have been changed to conceal the identities of patients and coworkers, and in the interest of protecting patient and staff confidentiality some characters are composites. Conversations and events in *The Shift* are reproduced to the best of my memory, though I have altered some short exchanges for clarity. The real patient behind the character of Ray Mason in *The Shift* gave me permission to tell his story here. HIPAA requirements make it potentially illegal for hospital nurses to track patients down after they've been discharged from the hospital and I did not attempt that for the other patients in this book. To avoid casting aspersions on a particular practice group I made up the incident where a procedure is done only because a patient requests it. Similar events have happened in the hospital, though. Finally, this book is not a medical textbook and should not be used as such: highly individual cases are discussed and are not necessarily suggestive of disease or treatment effects in the aggregate. All errors are my own.

CONTENTS

THE SHIFT

A Clean, Well-Lighted Place

The buzz of the alarm surprises me, as it always does. Six a.m. comes too soon. I've been off for a few days and never go to bed early enough before a first shift back. That's the problem with being a night owl at heart.

I lie in bed and think, What if I just don't go in today at all? I consider it, then realize how much the nurses I work with would hate me if I didn't show up.

I close my eyes one last time, though. It feels good to float in the warm darkness, Arthur, my husband, asleep next to me. There won't be any floating once I hit the hospital floor. I'll have drugs to deliver, intravenous lines to tend, symptoms to assess, patients in need of comfort, doctors who will be interested in what I have to say and others who won't, and my fellow RNs, who with a combination of snark, humor, technical skill, and clinical smarts, work, like me, to put our shoulders to the rock that is modern health care and every day push it up the hill.

The memory of that effort comes back to me, keeping me in bed, but there's something else, too, some feeling I don't want to own up to. It's why I'm hiding under the covers: I'm afraid. Afraid of that moment when the rock slips and all hell breaks loose.

For me it was the patient who started coughing up blood and within five minutes was dead, just like that. I've told the story many times, written about it, thought about it. Seven years later it has gotten easier. But remembering it I feel a flutter in my stomach, a tightening of my jaw.

That day the rock wrenched itself free, and until then I hadn't fully understood that we could completely lose control of a body in our care. It wasn't for lack of exertion; it was destiny, or fate if you prefer, that tore the rock away from me. I had run after it hard and fast, doing CPR in scrubs splattered with blood and calling in the code team—those professionals, usually from the ICU, trained for "rapid responses," who try to rescue patients when they crash. The nurses and doctors did their best for this patient, but they couldn't save her, and in the end a person who'd been alive and talking and laughing was living no more.

I put that memory away, get out of bed. It's early November and dark out and I prepare for Pittsburgh's late-autumn weather by pulling on riding tights and my wool sweater that proclaims "Ride Like a Girl." The sweater makes me feel young.

Brushing my hair, I almost forget to put on my necklace—a small silver heart charm surrounded by the words "I" and "Y-O-U." The heart has the tiniest of rubies stuck in the center, so that when it catches the light it seems to glow with life,

like a human heart. Arthur gave me the necklace for our an-
niversary a few years back. I reach behind my neck with both
hands and secure the clasp, comforted by having a reminder of
love in the hospital.

As I move down the stairs, the house is hushed. Arthur remains asleep, as do our three children. I think about the sleeping
kids, and a smile crosses my face: our son is fourteen, our twin
daughters, eleven, all with variations on their dad's curly hair,
the girls blond, as I used to be, too. None of them will get up for
school until long after I'm gone. The dog doesn't even wake up
with me in the morning, but the truth is, I like it quiet like this.
The warm blue of our cabinets and our pot rack in front of the
kitchen window make me happy. In the silence of the morning I
take a mental snapshot of the kitchen as a dose of home. Home
is a vaccine against the stresses of nursing.

Oh, food! I pick up a banana from our fruit bowl, peel it
fast, and then eat it while drinking a glass of water. I should
scramble eggs, toast bread, or even pour a bowl of cereal, but I
don't get up early enough to do any of that, and anyway I'm not
hungry first thing in the morning. My mother tells me my eating habits around work are unhealthy. *Uh-huh.* She's right, and
the irony is not lost on me, but the shift starts at 7:00 a.m. and
I'm never hungry until 9:00. I can't change that.

Lunch? I grab a yogurt, an apple, slap together a turkey
sandwich, light on the mayo, and stow it all in my bike bag. The
cafeteria food all tastes the same to me so I try not to buy my
lunch. I see my reflection in the glass sliding door. Don't have
my game face on yet: my blue eyes look wary, waiting. The house

remains silent as I sit on the stairs and tie my biking shoes. Then I put my bright yellow Gore-Tex jacket on, wrap my neck for warmth, and slide my bag over my shoulder.

I head down into what a friend calls our Norman Bates basement. It's where I keep my bike. There's no dead mother down here preserved with taxidermy, although you could find more than a few cobwebs and the sparse lighting makes the corners impenetrable. As a child I was terrified of the basement in our house and my best friend loved to tell stories about horrors befalling innocent young girls in creepy basements. I wonder why I listened to her. I must have enjoyed the thrill, that frisson of fear that came from transforming our very ordinary cellar into a place of the macabre.

My bike is stacked up against our family's four other bikes. The basement is limbo, a portal between the ordinary joys and struggles of home and the high-stakes world of the hospital. I put on my helmet and lock the basement door behind me as I leave, awkwardly carrying my bike out the low door and up the few steps. As usual, I'm running late. I turn on my bike lights, saddle up, and push off.

It's two miles to the hospital and the ride starts with a downhill. I enjoy the feeling of moving without work, having the world shoot past as I pick up speed, my front light illuminating a slim strip of road. I barely brake at the first stop sign, making a quick left down an even steeper hill that makes me go even faster. The rush is fun.

The next bit, mostly flat, gives me time to think. Like many nurses, the thing I'm always worried about is doing either too much or too little. If I sound an alarm and the patient is OK, then I over-reacted and have untrustworthy clinical judgment. If I don't call in the cavalry when it's needed, then I'm negligent and unsafe for patients. You don't always know because what goes on inside human bodies can be hidden and subtle. This job would be easier if there weren't such a narrow divide between being the canary in the coal mine and Chicken Little.

I push hard during the one small uphill on my way to the hospital, neck scarf up and over my mouth. The cold makes the passageways in my lungs constrict when they shouldn't, giving me that scary feeling of not being able to fully draw in a deep breath: bronchospasm. Covering my mouth and nose with a fleece wrap warms the air enough that I breathe just fine. I could carry an asthma inhaler, too, the medication that reopens those passageways, but that feels like overkill. At work I'll pump medicine costing $10,000 a bag into patients' veins, but use an inhaler? Me? That's for people who are sick.

There's not a hint of sunrise at the hospital parking lot, but cars scoot in and out of the gated entrance: the start of change of shift even though the day hasn't yet officially broken. I glide in around the barricade to the metal bike rack just inside the parking garage on my right.

In the parking lot nurses, doctors, patients, family, friends drive in expectant, worried, excited, hurting. They grip glowing cell phones, hard-to-read pagers, pieces of paper, extra clothing, all while waiting impatiently, anxiously, expectantly for the elevator.

The hospital itself is a paradox. Despite its occasional terrors, it is undeniably an oasis for the ill and infirm, a clean, well-lighted place. Sick people come, bringing their hopes and fears and we minister to them with our, mostly, good intentions.

That phrase "a clean, well-lighted place" comes from a Hemingway story. It's a short short story, about five pages long, in which, really, not much happens. The main character is a middle-aged waiter who works in a late-night café. He says some people require "a clean, well-lighted café" and late at night especially. Because of his own insomnia he understands why in the wee hours someone might need somewhere to go that's not home and not a bar.

But the young waiter he works with doesn't agree that the café needs to stay open so late. "Hombre, there are bodegas open all night long," he complains, eager to close up, go home, be with his wife.

"You do not understand," the older waiter says, "This is a clean and pleasant café. It is well lighted. The light is very good." It's two thirty in the morning and their one customer is an elderly man, a drunk who, the week before, tried to kill himself. If necessary, the older waiter will keep the café open all night to give sanctuary to this one forlorn soul.

However, his generosity to the patrons of the café stems not from compassion only, but his own hopelessness as well: "It was not fear or dread. It was a nothing that he knew too well. It was only that and light was all it needed and a certain cleanness and order." A feeling of dark disorder has overtaken him and he keeps the café open in part to keep his own nihilism at bay. But he also knows something the eager young waiter does not.

There will come a time when each of us will need a clean, well-lighted place that stays open all day and night, offering shelter from life's storms.

This is a hospital.

I work on a cancer ward, and while "cancer" used to always imply "death," more often than not that's not true anymore. Now, cancer involves treatment and its accompaniments: chemotherapy, radiation, surgery, scans, clinic visits, and hospital stays. People survive, often. We cure them—put their cancer into remission, forever one hopes—and they go home. Indeed, an oncology nurse's favorite words to a patient are, "I hope I never see you here again," and we're telling the truth.

The older waiter and I both come to work with the hope of doing good, and we share the same wish: for our customers, or patients, not to need us. But until that moment comes we will remain at our posts, ready.

AS I TAKE OFF MY GLOVES to lock up my bike, I shake my head. My friend Beth, another nurse at work, told me when she started this job she used to stop her car and vomit on the way to the hospital. I arrive with my heart racing from the bike ride, but the exercise also mellows my pre-work unease. Here I am, a forty-five-year-old mother of three with a PhD in English working as a nurse. People in health care—other nurses, doctors—weren't sure about me at first, thought I'd made a strange choice in choosing nursing over teaching. Now they're used to me. I show up and try hard; for everyone who counts, that seems to be enough.

The November cold nips at my bare hands as I walk toward the hospital, but as soon as I step inside the sliding glass entry doors blasts of warm air hit me. Sweat pricks on my back and I shimmy out of my bright yellow jacket, unzip my wool sweater, unwrap my neck, all while walking. I'm propelled by forward momentum and will stay that way for the entire twelve hours of my shift. It's good I work only three days a week. I live the other four days at a more normal pace.

A few nurses in white scrubs pass me on their way out and a few younger docs in white coats sleepily make their way down the hall ahead of me, their pockets bulging with folded papers. A surgeon I recognize steps out of the cafeteria gripping a paper cup of coffee from which he aggressively sips, though it's clearly steaming hot.

Two fresh-faced residents—new MDs in the middle of their on-the-job training—get on the same elevator I do, heads buried in their notes, talking excitedly in our shared language of medical acronyms, polysyllabic procedures, and body parts. An ICU nurse I'm friendly with steps on next, wearing the characteristic blue scrubs. A housekeeper carrying extra trash bags and a dry mop slides in just before the door closes.

"Hey," says Karla, the ICU nurse, as she looks me up and down, takes in my tights, the waterproof jacket hung over my arm. "You rode your bike today?"

"Uh-huh."

"Isn't it cold?" she grimaces.

"Not once I get moving."

"You're nuts," she says, waving as she steps off the elevator.

I laugh my loud laugh and wave back. Then she's gone.

Biking to the hospital gives me an unexpected patina of toughness, which matters in health care. Hospitals are filled with caring staff, but resilience and determination are prized as highly as empathy. In the vernacular, it comes down to whether someone's "got the balls" to make x, y, or z happen. The contrast between the empathy we're supposed to have and constant talk of "growing a set" or "who's got the cojones to . . ." can be jarring, but a big rock, no kidding, needs a nurse with the stones to move it.

I yawn, then chuckle to myself that a two-mile bike ride in the early winter cold hasn't woken me up. The housekeeper catches my eye as I yawn again. "I hear that," she says.

On my floor I change clothes in the general employee bathroom. We used to have a locker room with its own bathroom, but then they moved the locker room farther away, dolled it up, but forgot about a bathroom. I don't really care, except I get dressed for work in here and God only knows what killer microbes live on the floor, no matter how often they clean it.

My bike clothes come off and I pull on white scrubs, chilled and stiff from the ride. Done. I give my face a glance, just long enough to make sure I'm not sweaty. No makeup because, as a nurse I know says, "This is a dirty job." My necklace's reflection catches my eye in the mirror: O-U-Y ♥ I. I reach up and wrap my fingers around it. *Always*, I think.

Grabbing my bike clothes and bag, I pad in my sock feet into our redecorated (but less hospitable) staff locker room. I give my combination lock a few fast, practiced spins and pop open the door. Here I have everything I need to get through the next twelve hours: ink pen, flashlight, scissors, tape, blue IV caps, alcohol wipes, saline flushes, and a Sharpie. I stuff all that stuff into the different pockets of my scrubs and hang up my biking gear.

My bike shoes go onto a communal rack in a corner of the room and I slide into my nurse shoes with their thick soles. Leaving my work shoes at the hospital insures that hospital germs stay at work, too. I clip my ID badge onto my scrub top, completing the transformation from regular person to nurse. My lunch, such as it is, goes into our staff refrigerator and as I swipe my ID down our time clock's side channel I put on that game face while deliberately moving the pleasures and pulls of home to the back of my mind.

A shift lasts twelve hours. Twelve hours of holding a few lives in my hands, trying to make order out of the chaos of bodies and disease, working within a health care system that sometimes forgets it exists to serve human beings rather than bureaucrats or businessmen.

Amid the many uncertainties of the shift there is one thing I know for sure. Am I ready and up to the job? Yes. Today, and every day, for the sake of my patients I have no other option; the answer has to be, and always is, Yes.

CHAPTER 1

7:03am

I hit the floor at 7:03. It should be 7:00, but getting here almost late is my small, immature act of rebellion.

My very first clinical instructor told us, "If you're early, you're on time, and if you're on time, you're late." There was no "And if you're late . . ." Late being so catastrophic that its consequence couldn't even be spoken of. But here I am at the hospital, three minutes late, and nothing at all happens.

My eyes are wide, my muscles tense, but there's rarely any drama at the start of a morning shift. The floor is silent enough that my shoes make just the slightest squeak as I walk. In the hospital, if it's a good day, nothing much real happens before eight or nine a.m.

At the nurses' station the night-shift RNs cluster on chairs, looking like birds wanting to shove their tired heads under a free wing. Their lined faces and heavy-lidded eyes show how hard it is to stay awake and alert for an entire night. I don't work a lot of nights, but when I do I feel it. I hit a wall at 2:00 a.m., then again at 4:00. The hospital's strong tea, bad coffee, Diet Coke from the vending machine—they all help, but nothing non-pharmaceutical will really make me feel *awake* for the entire night, and I'm not going down the pharmacologic road. The day after, even if I sleep all morning and afternoon, it feels as though I'm seeing the world through gauze.

And yet there are compensations at night. It's calmer than daylight and watching over people as they sleep can be peaceful. Night is also when some patients plumb their deepest fears and talk about death, and paradoxically, in the darkness, the possibility of dying becomes less scary for some.

"How was the night?" I ask Linda, the nurse sitting closest to me at the nurses' station.

"Quiet," she says.

"Yeah, for you!" Melanie calls out, her eyes fixed on her computer.

I raise my eyebrows. "ICU transfer," Linda says.

"Who?" Not one of our familiar faces, I hope. We all get attached to certain patients and families. If one of them ends up in intensive care in the middle of the night that is not good news.

"New admission. We don't know him. Visiting family from Ohio."

"Ugh. That sucks. Talk about ruining your vacation."

"Yeah, the family was freakin' out, the guy's pressure was,

like, seventy over forty and he was just lying there drooling on himself." Melanie's turned toward me now. She raises her hands in a gesture of frustration.

"Is he OK?" I ask.

"Let me see—" she turns back to the computer and types something in, looking for him on the list of ICU patients. Some nurses believe that using the computer to follow patients in the hospital violates patient confidentiality laws, but I've never officially heard that, and so far no nurse I know has gotten reprimanded for it.

Melanie skims his electronic file. "Heart rate . . . blood pressure—Yes!—one hundred over sixty." She turns around to face me again.

I frown, thinking. "Sepsis?"

"No. He wasn't an onc. patient; they just didn't have a family practice bed."

"Whaddya think? Could he have just been dehydrated?"

"Well, probably not with that drooling!" She returns to the computer, intent on the paperwork—charting—she has to complete. The paperwork demands have steadily increased over time and the busier a nurse is with a very sick patient the more charting is required, even though she has less time to do it in. Computers should make the process faster, easier, but instead of efficiency, they enforce thoroughness. We're expected to chart almost everything, preferably in real time. Real time charting is impossible, though, if a patient needs a lot of immediate care.

I reach out for the printed papers I get for each of my patients and overhear another patient's name—Ray Mason—from a nearby conversation.

"What's Ray doing here?"

"Relapse," Helen, another night shift nurse who's walked over, says. Her mouth looks sour and she lets the single word hang in the air.

Dammit, I think, and then, "What?" Maybe if I pretend I don't understand what Helen has said it will make the fact of Ray's relapse untrue.

"Uh-huh," Helen says.

"When?" I ask.

She inclines her head. "Few days ago." She shrugs. Does it really matter? Nurses work a couple days on, a few days off, so we don't always hear the news. For me, ignorance helps maintain a border between home and the hospital.

"But I had coffee with him last month, him and Liz."

"I did the same," she says, "Except it was a beer."

Having coffee with a patient is unusual. Normally I would never meet a patient outside the hospital, but Ray was different. A firefighter who sings and plays guitar in a punk rock band is obviously an unusual combination. Ray's appeal, though, came from his easy way of being in the world and his unaffected bravery. We also had the same birthday, and when you work with cancer patients, that kind of coincidence ends up feeling significant.

Ray is young: twenty-five when he developed leukemia. He'd noticed himself growing daily more and more tired, and then he had a bruise that blossomed into a deep purple bulge under the skin of his lower abdomen. Something about its intensity and spread seemed unnatural. Next he caught a cold that, no matter what he did, just wouldn't go away.

The tiredness was what sent him to the doctor. Firefighters can't be chronically exhausted and Ray played hard, too: kids, the band, parties. The fatigue was making his job hard and cramping his style.

I see the coffee shop where we met in my mind's eye, at the bottom of one of the narrow slanted streets in Pittsburgh's Polish Hill neighborhood. Sunlight streamed in through big plate-glass windows. We'd cured his cancer and I asked Ray how he felt now that his disease was in remission. "The future looks brighter than bright," he told me. As he held up his hands, gesticulating, he seemed to hold the light between them. "Life," he said, "is better than it ever has been," and Liz, his wife, who was also there, agreed.

Time passed like liquid honey pouring out of a jar, slow and just sweet enough. People came and went from the coffee shop, wearing their own multi-zippered black leather jackets and worn T-shirts with combative slogans. Everyone knew Ray. "Hey, how you feeling?" was the most common question, with casual talk about music, where Ray's band was playing next. Around noon Ray ordered a sandwich and I got another latte. Liz stretched out her legs and asked what else I wanted to know, because they knew I was a writer and that their story captivated me.

I remember the creamy taste of my latte, the electric connection between the two of them, the crumbs of bright green spinach wrap left on Ray's plate, the future hanging pendulous, infinite. In this moment I thought that Ray would stay healthy forever. He would work, raise his children, grow old, and die when the time was right, but not before. He would fight fires and save lives and he and Liz would keep looking toward the future, drawn in by its promise.

I believed it. I believed that meeting outside the hospital and talking only of a rosy what-would-be could conjure a permanent remission. I believed it, when I knew that, for better and for worse, time never stops for long.

Relapse—the return of disease—is not unlikely for patients with Ray's kind of leukemia, but I'm shocked that he's back on the floor. I'm also angry, really angry. And then I pull myself back to my work.

"Do I have Ray?" I ask Helen, the night-shift nurse. She was officially in charge overnight, making her the "charge nurse": a bedside RN who functions as a manager for that particular shift. Charge nurses—also called resource nurses at some hospitals—assign patients to staff, troubleshoot, and perform set administrative tasks, such as making sure the crash cart (a toolbox of equipment and drugs we need in an emergency) is ready to go. Some RNs bowdlerize "charge nurse" to "charge bitch" because for the wrong kind of person it becomes a power trip, but Helen's not like that.

She shakes her head—Ray will not be mine today—and I am relieved. I prefer to be Ray's nurse later, not right now when cancer once again has the early advantage, before we've put our own treatment plan into motion

I pick up the papers for my patients, fingering them with

the contained apprehension of a poker player gathering in a hand on which she's already bet more than she can afford. The patients are the key to the entire shift: they can make a day intolerably frustrating or unbelievably rewarding, or occasionally both. For each patient there are two pages of information stapled together and those pages tell me their names, birth dates, medications, diet orders, trends in lab values, and a brief medical history, which oddly enough is not always correct. For the moment I ignore all that detail and start by learning who these people are.

Tense, but also curious, I read the names to myself: Richard Hampton, Dorothy Sooth, and Sheila Field. Dorothy I know, the other two I don't. Skimming the papers I pull out the most basic information. Richard Hampton is a lymphoma patient in his late seventies. Dorothy Sooth, a cheerful woman who keeps a well-stocked candy dish in her room, is in her late fifties and was hospitalized for the initial treatment of her leukemia. Everyone knows Dorothy, who is getting to the end of her six-week stay. My third patient, Sheila Field, in her midforties, came in with a blood clotting disorder called antiphospholipid antibody syndrome. It sounds intriguing.

I look at Helen, eyebrows raised, "Three?" I ask, with a half-smile.

"Well, yeah," she says. "You've got that empty room between A15 and A17, but there're no scheduled admissions today."

"Sweet."

"Of course, if someone comes in . . ."

"Right—they'll be mine. I'll enjoy it while it lasts," I tell her.

The difference between three and four patients is huge. Three to four is supposed to be a standard load and that usually ends up being four, but there are no official rules about how many patients we can have. If we're working short-staffed four patients will jump to five and night shift occasionally has six each.

There are stem cell transplant units where each nurse covers only two patients—the ideal level of care for our sickest people. With four patients they sometimes become human to-do lists and I could get a fourth anytime: a transfer from intensive care, an admission from the Emergency Department, someone with a new diagnosis of leukemia jerked out of his normal life and pulled, unwilling, into the world of the hospital. This unknown fourth patient feels like a vulture perching on my shoulder, hungry to scavenge my peace of mind, so I try not to think about it.

Three allows me to treat my patients as people. Instead of rushing from room to room I can move at a human pace and also be on top of everything going on with them: talking to worried family members who call, knowing the results of recent scans and tests so that I can answer questions knowledgeably, tuning in to iffy vital signs, or pushing a physician to come up with an anti-nausea regimen for a patient who's spent two solid days vomiting.

Hospital administrators with their eyes on the bottom line seem to think that nurses can stretch infinitely, like rubber bands. The fewer the number of nurses the lower the labor costs for the hospital. But if I give care a numerical value, represented by TLC, while P stands for number of patients and RN for each individual nurse, then:

$$\frac{RN}{p} = TLC$$

The more patients an individual nurse cares for, the smaller the amount of TLC per patient. More significantly, research on staffing levels has made it pretty clear that the more patients a nurse has above a certain number (the number itself depends on the patient population and how sick the patients are), the larger the likelihood a patient will die who wouldn't have otherwise. In other words, nurse-to-patient ratios aren't just about patients feeling cared for; they're also about fragile people staying alive.

Of course administrators have their own different formula with KVIs—Key Volume Indicators—and FTEs—full-time employees. My eyes glaze over when I try to understand health care economics from a manager's point of view. I say, put the patient at the center and figure out the money from there.

I pick up the portable phone that night-shift left out for me and idly clean it with one of the packaged alcohol wipes I keep in my scrub pockets. Every floor has its own supply of phones and each nurse is assigned one for the day. There aren't enough for each of us to have our own permanent one. They are expensive, but often don't work well, probably because they are accidentally dropped over and over during the day. They all also have identical ring tones, so when one phone goes off we all have to pull out our own to discover whose it actually is. By the end of shift there's a ringing in my head that only time away from work can dim the sound of.

The phone is a mercurial presence on the job. The calls always have a claim of urgency, so I'll answer if I'm eating or even if I'm changing a dressing on a wound. I could have just buttonholed a doctor who's notoriously hard to pin down only to have him scurry off when my phone rings. Wherever I am, if my phone rings I will probably answer it because, more often than seems possible, I really do need to know what the person calling has to say.

Every nurse I know has at one time or another wanted to throw her phone against a wall or casually, as if by accident, drop it out a window. If I did that, though, the charge nurse would just get me another one, so I slide it into a pocket of my scrubs.

Once when I was a new nurse I got an aide's phone by accident. It was the only phone left in the drawer and looked just like one of ours. The problem was, it couldn't receive calls from outside the hospital and no one told me, so the doctor I'd been paging about a patient's chest pain never called me back, or rather, did call me back from his own off-site clinic, but couldn't reach me. We called in a rapid response team—the people who come when a patient seems to be taking a serious turn for the worse—and that patient spent the night in intensive care, "just in case." All of that drama and activity might have been avoided if I'd had the right phone.

I check my watch. It's 7:15 and I'm already behind. This half hour, from 7:00 to 7:30, is when I organize my day. I put my papers in order based on room number and pull a blank sheet out of the computer printer tray and staple it on top for notes. Electronic health records are ubiquitous in health care, but in the hospital we remain dependent on our physical "papers."

I fold the blank sheet of paper into fourths. Then I take my pen and outline the four squares I just made by drawing along the fold. Each patient gets one square and I have a blank square for the fourth patient if she or he shows up. I number each square at the top with the patient's room number and write in each patient's name. Then I draw the grids we use to write down laboratory values and add in the abbreviations for intravenous lines. So strange to me as a new nurse, these now come easily. TLHC is a triple lumen Hickman catheter, a permanent IV line that protrudes from the upper chest. A PICC—peripherally inserted central catheter—is a different type of permanent IV line that gets inserted in the patient's upper arm. Temporary IVs I notate as "per," because they go into a peripheral vein: the kind you can see when you look at your own arm or hand.

I used to need a full sheet of paper for each patient, but now it's one 4.25" x 5.5" square of white each. I've got my printed papers, too, of course, that come from the computer, but this one-sheet documentation of the day is uniquely mine. It's just enough space, I hope, to record all the variables of the shift, including the new information I cannot forget: an MD called to consult when a patient will go off the floor for a scan, a cell phone number from a distraught husband or wife, the specific bacteria found growing in culture, test results whether good or bad, and new orders from the nurse practitioners, physician assistants, or MDs.

If it's a bad day, I'll know because that small quarter of a page of white paper won't be big enough for everything I need to write down.

CHAPTER 2

Report

The other day-shift nurses, like me in white scrubs, are already in the conference room. I see Amy, with her long blond hair, and Katherine, one of our veteran nurses who actually works two jobs. Their form of rebellion is wearing colored long-sleeve shirts under their white scrub tops.

Susie, one of our newer nurses, is there and her tight curls bob as she nods her head and writes. I know Randy, also a newer nurse, is on today, but he likes to go somewhere quiet for report. Quiet can be good, but today I want the social connection.

There's Nora, who can be a great coworker, but has a catty side I don't much like, and Dot, whose throaty smoker's laugh inexplicably comforts me; not much throws Dot.

And last I see my friend Beth, who's maybe ten years older than I am and stopped throwing up on her way to work a long time ago. Her hair is cut just above her shoulders in a tidy, middle-aged bob. Her wire-rimmed glasses flash up at me as she offers me a wave and a smile, but she doesn't stop listening and writing.

This is what we call "report." The nurses all sit, intent, portable phones up to their ears, writing down histories, numbers of white blood cells, chemotherapy regimens, problems we've yet to solve. It's an internal room, windowless. A half-full two-liter bottle of Diet Coke, a leftover from night shift, or who knows when, sits out on the table along with some stacked Styrofoam cups. The soda's probably flat, but I bet at some point today someone will drink it anyway.

Listening to voice care can be a little like attending a spoken-word poetry slam. Near the end of every shift each nurse uses the phone to tape a verbal report on each of her or his patients. Report always begins with the same information: name, age, diagnosis, but after that every nurse has her own style, her own points of emphasis. We're people after all and some nurses will discuss the most pressing issues first, while other nurses describe all the normals before getting into what's really up. With cancer patients, in general, something is always up. Plus, some nurses like to know everything about a patient, others the bare minimum, and the report we give reflects our own inclinations. Katherine is notorious for reports that come across like haikus. Beth tends toward the epic. I try to be concise, then catch myself rambling; later I'll worry that some important detail got left out because of my self-editing.

Report is also always in our unique hospital lingo, which includes acronyms and diagnoses, but explains events in terms of well-known clinical narratives:

"Lisa Smith, you know her, day ten of a MUD, intractable nausea and vomiting. We're trying Ativan and it seems to be working, but knocks her out." Translation: the tenth day after her matched unrelated donor transplant.

"Bob Jones has a fungal pneumonia. He just couldn't stop smoking and we can't give ampho because he's allergic to it." Amphotericin B is a potent but toxic antifungal medication.

"Diane Doe, day twenty-four of an Auto and . . . let me look it up . . . her ANC is, oh my God, her ANC is already back and it's eight hundred. She's going home." ANC is absolute neutrophil count, a measure of immune system function.

Voice care is efficient. In the old days report was given from nurse to nurse face-to-face, which took all the nurses off the floor at the same time. With voice care the shift going off duty covers while the shift coming on duty listens, but nuances get lost on the tape. A grimace, raised eyebrows, a frown communicate the feel of taking care of someone. Voice care passes on the details of a patient's stay, but it doesn't always capture who the patient is.

Some hospitals are starting to do change of shift with both nurses in the room talking to each other and the patient. The idea is to make the patient a partner in care and to smooth out the transition between nurses. I like the sound of it, just as I agree with letting patients read their own medical records, but what about the patients who consciously choose to know only the broad outlines of their care because hearing all the details makes them anxious? Treatment for cancer is not like having your gallbladder removed; some patients want to know everything, while others prefer to remain as ignorant as possible. And sometimes we keep secrets from patients, usually when the news is bad and we want to be 100 percent sure before confirming it. Will a face-to-face report lead to all patients learning new medical information in real time, or will we sometimes deliberately hide what we know, institutionalizing a layer of deception? Knowledge is power, but how much and when for each individual patient?

Then there are the petty secrets nurses want to keep among ourselves: that we find a patient whiny, that his wife is suspicious of everything we do, that the relatives who visit expect us to chat with them, making it impossible to get any work done. Should complaints be part of report? Underneath the fog of irritation, venting can reveal the human being. But maybe being in the room with the real patient would be an even better reminder of her humanity.

I dial up voice care and punch in my access code, pen ready. I have to go fast.

I hear Andie, the night-shift nurse, telling me about my patients. When one nurse's patients get transferred as a group to another, as happened this morning for me, report is easier. That kind of easy pass isn't always possible, though, since the number of staff and patients can vary. Richard Hampton, the seventy-five-year-old with lymphoma, is having some difficulty breathing and is off and on confused. In other words, he's elderly, has cancer, and is not doing so well. I scribble down how his night was. No alarming highs or lows in his daily lab reports—also called lab values or just labs, for short—that we need to address, but I'm not sure what, if anything, we'll be able to do for him. The printout I got lists his meds, but Andie doesn't mention a treatment plan. Seems like, except for his cancer, the fact that he can't breathe without oxygen, and doesn't always know where he is, he's doing great. I sigh inwardly—cancer sucks, it really does—and punch in the number for my second patient.

Next up is Dorothy Webb, beloved by everyone because she's very friendly and because of that candy dish in her room, located right next to the door. Dorothy, fifty-seven, came in with leukemia, went into remission after chemo, and now we're keeping her until her immune system returns close enough to normal that it's safe for her to go home. For the next several months she'll come back to the hospital every few weeks for what we call consolidation chemo: high-dose chemotherapy to help maintain her remission. None of that's on the table today, though; today she's mostly waiting, stir-crazy, I learn, but from an illness point of view doesn't have a lot going on.

Sheila Field, my third patient, is a wild card. She arrived at three this morning from an outside hospital and I learn that she's got a history of a blood clotting disorder—ah, that's the "antiphospholipid antibody syndrome."

Sheila puts the "heme" in hematology/oncology, which is what our floor specializes in. Blood disorders like hers and blood cancers such as leukemia and lymphoma are both considered problems of hematology, the study of how blood is produced and what its diseases are. Blood cancers are also categorized under "oncology," the same as solid-tumor cancers (such as lung, breast, liver), and some clinicians even describe leukemia and lymphoma as "liquid tumors." For me, Sheila provides a break from cancer and a chance to learn. I, too, forget that "heme/onc," as we describe ourselves, includes blood disorders of all stripes. Blood seems so simple—a cut bleeds and then clots, red blood cells carry oxygen—but there are people whose blood itself is dangerously flawed and Sheila may be one of them.

I click the phone off and glance over my notes; everything looks OK. The clock on the wall says 7:30. I need to find Andie; she'll be wanting to go home to sleep.

She's waiting at the nurses' station. Young and pretty, her thick black hair piled up on her head, her delicate neck bent with fatigue, she looks like a drooping flower.

"Any updates?"

"Naaw," she says, trying to stifle a yawn. "Dorothy's ANC isn't back yet." That's her Absolute Neutrophil Count: a specific type of white blood cell crucial for fighting infections. It's Dorothy's neutrophils that have to regrow enough for her to go home. "This guy, Richard Hampton, I don't know what they're gonna do with him."

"Is there a plan?"

"Not that I've heard," she says.

"Anything else on Sheila?"

"God, you know, did they really have to bring her here in

the middle of the night? They couldn't just let her sleep?" she asks. I used to underestimate Andie because of her looks. Stupid. She's a damn good nurse.

"Well, it's the old 'Send 'em to Pittsburgh; they'll know what to do,'" I say.

She frowns. "Yeah, right."

"Go home," I tell her.

She nods, looks down at her notes one last time. "Oh, wait, she's also having some belly pain."

"Abdominal pain?"

"Yep. Not too too bad, but it hurts."

I purse my lips, wrinkle my eyebrows. Could be any number of things.

I nod. "See ya," I say, as she slowly walks away, yawning again, this time not trying to hide it.

In the hospital, this is friendship. We take a "just the facts, ma'am" approach, and add in an ineffable bit more. "Only connect," the novelist E. M. Forster famously wrote. "Go home," I tell Andie, in place of saying how much I admire her and wish her well. No time for any of that right now.

I look up at the whiteboard across the nurses' station from me. It's got twenty-eight rows delineating our twenty-eight rooms and they're all numbered and divided into sections. The first three letters of each patient's last name go in the blank space following the room number—laws about patient confidentiality forbid us from writing more. The next space lists the attending physician. This is the doctor who has ultimate responsibility for the patient and supervises morning rounds but will not be physically in the hospital during the day to address problems. That work—daily medical care—is done by interns and residents, nurse practitioners, and physician assistants, and their names go in the empty space following the attending physician's.

In any teaching hospital, interns and residents are completing the intense clinical training that follows their four years of medical school. They are technically already doctors, but residency is when they really learn how to be doctors. Internship is the first year of residency and so first-years are called "interns." After that they become "residents." For them, this is the time of no sleep and being "pimped": asked questions so persistently by attending physicians on rounds that even the most prepared intern eventually runs out of answers. In the end she may feel foolish and exposed, but also by butting up against her own ignorance she will have learned something important—that's the idea at least. Most of the residents are nice, but some aren't; many understand how to work well with other people while others don't. They are trying awfully hard and many, especially in the first few months of each training year, seem anxious to do well.

First-year interns are supervised by residents, who in turn are supervised by older residents and fellows—MDs specializing in a field. The residents on my floor will become a variety of doctors, but the fellows are all "heme/onc." Nurse practitioners (NPs) and physician assistants (PAs) have many of the privileges and responsibilities of physicians, but most don't get paid close to a physician's salary. From what I've seen, inpatient care would collapse without them. They, similar to the interns and residents, do a lot of the daily medical work in the hospital.

True to tradition, the NPs and PAs are listed on the board by their first names, as nurses are, and the interns and residents by last names only. Any good history of medicine would have to examine how important the title "Dr." is to many MDs and how certain types of docs don't allow anyone but another doc to call them by their first name. That kind of attitude is changing in the newer generation; they tend to introduce themselves as "Lisa" or "John." But there are even now nurses who call every physician—whether an attending physician or intern—"Doctor" because that's how they were trained and what they believe is right.

I bring my informality to work as well as my background in a university. When I taught at Tufts I was Theresa and my husband is Arthur at the University of Pittsburgh physics department. Hierarchies in naming reinforce hierarchies of power and I guess that explains the rigidity about who's called what in hospitals, but health care might run more smoothly if those of us who work together used first names, identifying ourselves to each other at least as more equal than not.

The last two rows on the white board show the nurse's name and phone number. I pull out my phone and check the number taped to the back of it. Yes, they wrote it down correctly. Occasionally the numbers get mixed up and it's very confusing until someone figures out what happened and fixes it on the board.

I write down the pager numbers for my patients' clinicians (intern, NP, or PA), which I get from the other big white board we have. That board, hanging on a wall perpendicular to the first, includes key phone numbers: the blood bank, our satellite pharmacy, the lab, escort, MDs whose clinics are separate from the hospital, and so on.

Report done and all needed contact information written down, we nurses scatter to our pods and medcarts, compact wheeled sets of drawers that hold supplies and patients' medications and have a computer and work space on top. The top surface is higher than a normal desk so our chairs feel like barstools. If only.

I'm in the back part of the floor today, behind a set of double doors that keep the hallway pretty quiet, although they serve a practical purpose: protecting our stem cell transplant patients, who are particularly vulnerable to infections. The doors keep random visitors out and remind the patients not to mingle.

I sit down to do computer work and every nurse on the floor is doing essentially the same thing: looking up each patient's lab values, medication times, vital signs, and new orders. Then browsing the patient's history, checking test results, and confirming conclusions from scans. This is in some ways the most important part of the entire shift because it's when we prepare for the next eleven hours.

Looking up from my computer, I see Ray Mason's wife, Liz, farther down the hall, taking clean linens out of the cupboard. We're not supposed to let family members do this. It's considered an infection risk, which matters since so many of our patients are immune-suppressed, but some people can't tolerate feeling useless—they like to do for themselves—so I don't act as an enforcer. I'm here to care for people, not make them follow the rules, especially considering how often the rules around here change.

I walk over to Liz and we hug silently. I want to say something helpful, comforting, but she and I both know there's nothing good to say.

"It sucks, huh?" She nods and her eyes look wet. "How are you doing?"

She shrugs. "He's fine," she says, her voice lifting up at the end, implying that she's not. She hugs the sheets, blankets, and pillowcases to her chest and shakes her head. "He needs these," she says.

"Are you here today?" I ask.

"No, I . . . " she stops and her eyes squinch up. "My office says if I don't come in I could lose my job."

"But . . . they were so supportive before."

"Yeah," she inclines her head, compresses her lips. "I'm sure it will work out eventually." I think about her clients. She's a therapist who specializes in obsessive behaviors, so the people in her care are in need, too. But can she help them if she's focused on her husband, back in the hospital, once again fighting cancer? That's the hard thing about empathy—even people with an abundance of it can run out.

I grab her arm, wishing I weren't so powerless to help. Relapse typically leads to a stem cell transplant—Ray will need cells donated by someone else—and the choice is pretty much transplant or death, so almost everyone who can chooses transplant, but it's not an easy road. "In the midst of life we are in death," the Episcopal *Book of Common Prayer* says, reminding us that life is a continuum and we're all mortal. In my work with cancer patients I have found that the specter of death powerfully connects us to life. Maybe if I had Ray today I would have felt newly enlightened about my work as an oncology nurse, but it wasn't meant to be. "I'll come by," I say. She nods and we each head back to our own corner of the floor.

I check my watch: 8:20. I have time to look up antiphospholipid antibody syndrome. Google is where I would normally start and I can do that if I don't run into trouble with the filters on the computers. Nurses' access to online material is restricted, typically without notice. So one day I was denied admission to our online medical library. Another time I was blocked from chemoregimens.com, a website we use to double-check treatment protocols. It's frustrating to be restricted from knowledge, but it's humiliating to be trusted with the daily care of people who have life-threatening conditions and not be trusted with the level of Internet access required to learn about their problems. I can push doxorubicin, a drug that will burn skin and can damage hearts, into a patient's vein through an IV, but I'm not mature enough to use Google without filters designed for children?

We're told the filters were put in place to keep nurses from using social websites at work and in general to keep nurses from surfing the Web when we should be working. I don't honestly know if that's an issue. Maybe it is. All I can say is that no nurse I know wastes time on the Internet when there's work to be done.

Today, though, I'm allowed access to the information I need: antiphospholipid antibody syndrome is an autoimmune disease, like Lupus. It can occur secondary to an existing auto-immune disorder, but for other people (and my patient Sheila Field seems to be one of them) it arises on its own. Patients with this syndrome generate a mistaken immune response to crucial components of what's called the clotting cascade. Short version: their blood clots too easily.

It's essential to have blood clot when we're cut, saving our lives, but a blood clot inside the body, in an artery or vein where we need it to flow continuously, is damaging and potentially deadly. During a heart attack a clot blocks the blood supply to the heart muscle itself, causing part of the heart to die due to an absence of blood. Because cell death hurts, patients having heart attacks complain of crushing chest pain. The pain is the scream of all those cardiac cells dying.

I don't know if Sheila's heart or any other part of her body is at risk from her illness. I only learned about her stomach pain from Andie, so if that's part of the complete clinical picture, I'm not sure how it fits in. Judging by the paucity of the notes on her case it seems as though no one else has a clear picture of her situation either. I frown. It looks as if I'll have to wait until rounds to learn more.

I am clicking around more computer screens, writing down what I need, when the door to Richard Hampton's room opens and the intern (I think) walks out. His round glasses with thick frames make him appear owlish and though he's young, his hair is already thinning on top, adding to the impression that he's old before his time.

"Hey," I say quietly, giving a small wave.

"Are you his nurse?" he asks. His voice is soft and low and he bends in toward me. He looks so serious I can't imagine him smiling, but I like the intensity since I can be intense at work myself.

I nod at him, say my name.

He nods back, and then speaks again, very quietly and calmly. "So, it looks like we're going to give him Rituxan today," he says.

"Rituxan?" I ask, raising my eyebrows.

His features collapse and his face goes blank, a mask. "We'll discuss it on rounds, but the attending wants him to get Rituxan."

He grimaces, then walks away, but I feel my stomach tightening. Rituxan is a first-line treatment for certain lymphomas. It's not chemotherapy per se, but a biological response modifier, a drug that activates the patient's own immune system to kill cancer cells. For many people it's safe, but it has killed patients while being used correctly. Too much of an immune response can make a person very, very sick rather than well. In fact, that's often how influenza kills—it's not the virus itself that's deadly, but the overwhelming immune response it provokes.

Because of its potential dangers, Rituxan comes with a label reserved for particularly toxic drugs called a Black Box warning. That is, in addition to listing all possible side effects of the drug the information with Rituxan includes the most serious reactions inside a literal box drawn with thick, black lines. The Black Box warning for Rituxan includes death.

Bad diseases seem to require bad drugs and Rituxan is hardly the scariest of the treatments we use against cancer. Doctors even consider it "well-tolerated" and comparatively benign, because once it has been infused there are no long-term side effects. That allows it to be safely prescribed to seventy- and eighty-year-old patients who likely wouldn't survive the toxicities of more standard chemotherapies. If anyone asked me I would recommend Rituxan because it works for lymphoma patients, but nurses dislike giving it because infusing the drug doesn't always go well and we're responsible for keeping patients safe.

I watch the intern walk down the hall, slightly stooped, as if he bears the weight of the world on his shoulders. But it is I who will give Mr. Hampton his Rituxan, who will monitor him for serious changes in blood pressure, heart rate, and breathing, who will need to call this intern, or his replacement, if the treatment intended to heal ends up hurting instead. The intern doesn't know this drug as well as I do. The intern won't be the person hooking it up to Mr. Hampton's IV, watching it run down the plastic tubing directly into his vein, knowing that if things go badly it will be a result of the work of my own hands. And now I'm nervous. From what I've heard about Mr. Hampton's frailty, I'm worried he'll be particularly vulnerable to the rigors of Rituxan, that giving him this drug is a really bad idea. Before I become too committed to this line of thought, though, I decide to see Mr. Hampton for myself.

His room is dark, with just a hint of sun lightening the edges of the window blinds. He's on three liters of oxygen and it makes a subtle whistling sound that's not unpleasant.

"Mr. Hampton." I gently shake his shoulder to check for myself how responsive he is when awake. I would rather not wake him up, but there's no other way to find out and it's important. "I'm Theresa. I'm your nurse today."

He opens his eyes and looks at me blankly. "Do you know where you are?" It's a standard question for the confused. He blinks, but says nothing, then lies back on the bed while his eyes slowly shut.

Being awakened from a deep sleep would only make any confusion worse, but I've been told he's slept most of the time he's been in the hospital. That's not normal. He's thin and his face is lined and his white hair stands up in a peak over his brow. It is a shock of hair.

I decide to let him sleep and leave, shutting the door quietly behind me.

Then, worried about what the Rituxan might do to this old man, I start to blame the doctor for clinical myopia, for focusing on the need to treat without also considering the possibility of harm. Mr. Hampton is weak and breathing with difficulty. Can he tolerate this toxic drug?

The attending physician on this case is one of those docs who never discusses his decisions with anyone; he decides and the rest of us—interns and nurses both—do as he says. He could be right in ordering Rituxan for Mr. Hampton; that's not my call. For some patients it is a killing drug, but it's much better at getting rid of cancer cells than hurting people. All I want is a minute, maybe two, to confirm that the treatment isn't more harmful than curative, or if it is, that the patient or someone who can speak for him deems the risk worth it.

"Work is love made visible. And what is it to work with love?" the poet Khalil Gibran wrote. In the hospital, working with love sometimes requires putting people in danger. For Richard Hampton, my patient now destined for Rituxan, old, frail, and short of breath, we will try to save him by administering a drug that could end his life. That's a surprising kind of love, but in here it's very real.

For myself I wonder, will I kill this patient today or heal him? I'd like to have an idea of the specific degree of risk involved instead of relying on this queasy feeling in my gut. I look at my watch. It's 8:35. Even without talking it over, I'll find out soon enough if my gut is right.

CHAPTER 3

Hitting the Floor

Susie, the newbie, walks by me holding up a clear plastic bag filled with a thick, orangey fluid. "Have time to check platelets?" She's bright-eyed, overtly friendly, and those characteristics, combined with her blond curls, give her a Shirley Temple vibe. But the hospital is not the good ship *Lollipop*, not even close.

I nod. "Platelets so early in the morning?" Blood products usually don't get ordered until after the doctors' finish rounds.

We start to walk down the hall, toward her pod. "He's getting a line placed and they want him above fifty."

"Listen to you," I say, "slingin' the lingo." She smiles. Her patient needs an intravenous line surgically inserted and the surgeon putting in the line wants the patient's platelet count—platelets are the cells that cause blood to clot—to be 50,000 or greater. Otherwise there's a risk of bleeding. A normal number of platelets is 150,000 to 300,000, but in the hospital people will do OK with just 10,000, which is kind of unbelievable to me, but 10,000 platelets isn't enough if we're deliberately cutting into someone.

Susie's patient has the opposite problem from my patient Sheila. Sheila's blood clots when it shouldn't; because this patient's platelet count has been greatly reduced by chemotherapy, he probably won't clot when he needs to. Imagine a garden hose with no shut-off valve, except it's not water that can't be stopped from flowing out; it's human blood trickling from a vein. That's what life is like for hemophiliacs, and it is one of the dangers of cancer treatment. The platelet count will return to normal once treatment stops, but until that happens, giving patients platelets intravenously is the only way to replenish their supply. When we transfuse platelets two nurses first verify that the identification codes on the blood product and the patient match. That's what's required when "checking platelets."

We get to Susie's medcart and an older woman with short gray hair and a friendly face peers out of the partially opened door to one of the rooms. "Susie, do you mind coming to disconnect him? You know how he is about getting his morning shower."

Susie bites her lip. She needs to get the platelets in before her patient getting the IV line is called to surgery.

"I'll do that," I tell her. "You type in the numbers for the platelets and we'll check them after I've disconnected him from his IV."

"Really?"

"Sure."

"OK, thanks." She pulls up the right screen on our electronic record system and I head into the first patient's room, pulling out a wrapped saline syringe while I go.

"Hi, I'm Theresa. I'm helping Susie out." I squirt Purell from the dispenser on the wall into my hands and rub them together until it evaporates. Then I grab a pair of latex gloves and pull them on. Purell then gloves is the procedure we're supposed to follow and it's a rule I try to obey.

The gray-haired woman nods to me. "You girls are so busy I hate to ask for anything, but he's just a bear without his morning shower." This last bit she says in a mock whisper, hiding her mouth behind an exaggeratedly raised hand.

The gray-haired man in the bed speaks up now. "I'm a bear, am I? Well, you're a tiger without your morning coffee."

The woman laughs. "That's true, honey, but I can go and get my coffee myself. I don't have to be unhooked from this stupid machine."

"Ain't that the truth," he says. He's moved to the edge of the bed and I bend over his chest to follow his IV line to the red-tipped channel of his Hickman catheter, which protrudes from his right upper chest. The Hickman has three separate tube-like openings called lumens that hang down, so we call this a triple-lumen catheter. I stop his pump and then unscrew the IV from the Hickman, carefully putting a sterile red plastic cap that I have already taken out of my pocket and unwrapped on the end of the IV. Then I rub an alcohol wipe across the top of the lumen and push in the entire contents of the saline flush

I also just took out of its wrapper. This is standard procedure to keep the line free of germs and flowing smoothly.

"Do you need me to tape that up for you?" I ask. Our IV lines are covered with bandages, and we protect them with water-repellant plastic covers when patients take showers. A wet dressing offers a prime breeding ground for unwanted bacteria.

"Oh, no," the woman says. "We've developed our own system using Press 'n Seal."

"It's amazing I have any hair left on my chest!" the husband calls out to me as I turn to leave, but he's laughing as his wife approaches him with the plastic wrap.

Welcome to twenty-four-hour visiting. Family members sleep over, share meals, tease, bicker, joke, and sometimes evolve their own ways of doing things that make their lives, and ours, easier.

Susie's not in the hallway, but I see her in the other patient's room, helping him onto a stretcher that a technician from the operating room is steering. The technician's dressed in that blue-gray the OR staff wear, her hair protected by a filmy cover.

I poke my head in. "What's going on?"

"They're ready for him," Susie says, "Said to send the platelets down with the tech," she nods toward the woman holding the stretcher, "and they'll hang them." That is, the OR nurses will begin and monitor the platelet transfusion. "He got two bags already overnight so he should be good." She says "good" definitively and gives her patient an encouraging smile.

"Works for me. See ya."

I get back to my pod and the light above Sheila's doorway

turns on. I also hear the chime that goes with it. At this point in the shift it sounds soothing, melodic. By the end of the day I will be desperate to silence that ringing. Now, though, it's a gentle calling and I feel fresh, ready to be needed.

Sheila's my puzzle and I want to understand her disease better. The human clotting mechanism is an impressively complex series of chemical processes appropriately called a cascade. Something as simple as a paper cut activates two unique pathways of proteins called factors, which trigger a chemical called prothrombin, which becomes thrombin, and then activates fibrinogen, which turns into fibrin. Fibrin threads form the physical structure of a blood clot by giving platelets something to adhere to and thereby stop active bleeding. An error along any of these pathways can cause poor clotting or, as with Sheila, blood that clots too easily. It's one of those proverbial "for want of a nail" situations, where the lack of a nail for a horse's shoe leads to an undelivered message, a lost battle, and a vanquished kingdom. Every step of the human clotting cascade has to work correctly for the patient's blood to coagulate the way it should.

I'm sure Sheila's exhausted from her middle-of-the-night ambulance ride, so if she's turned on the call light this early in the morning it must be important.

Each pod on the floor has four rooms and the door to every room is usually kept shut to maintain a positive air pressure that stops any hallway germs from accidentally drifting inside and making one of our immune-suppressed patients sick; if the doors stay open for too long they trigger an alarm that penetrates like an aural jackhammer. The closed doors keep my patients safe from foreign contaminants, but at the same time keep me from quickly looking in and physically seeing how they're doing.

I push on Sheila's heavy door, trying to be quiet with the metal latch even though I know she couldn't have put on the call light if she weren't already awake. Her room is dark and she's buried—head and all—under a double layer of blankets. "Sheila? I'm Theresa, your nurse today." A hand edges out from beneath the blankets and I walk up to the bed after once again disinfecting my hands with Purell and grabbing a pair of gloves.

"Hurts." she says, in a high-pitched voice, pinched at the end, the volume muffled by her blankets.

"Your belly?"

"Hurts," she says again, and I see a nodding motion under the covers.

"I'll get you something for the pain," I tell her. That is one of my favorite hospital euphemisms: I'll get you *something* for the pain. Perhaps a mug of hot cocoa, a plush toy bunny with floppy ears, a warm compress delivered with a cool and gentle hand. No, *something* in this case refers to narcotics: Vicodin, oxycodone, Dilaudid, morphine. We give out these drugs like candy on Halloween; our patients need them.

Outside Sheila's room I run into the oncology fellow—an MD specializing in cancer, on his way to becoming an oncology attending—who's getting ready to go in himself. This fellow is kind and quite smart but hesitates over even the smallest decisions. I'm never sure if that's because he lacks confidence, or because his English is poor, or because he is genuinely interested in having a nurse's input. Let's hope it's reason number three.

"Yong Sun," I say, and get his wide friendly smile that makes his eyes crinkle up. "She's having abdominal pain—"

"Ahh, right," he interrupts. "Hmmmmm." He purses his lips. "What you think?"

"Not sure. But she doesn't have anything ordered for pain. You OK with Dilaudid IV?"

"Ah. Hmmm. Yes. One-time dose of Dilaudid, 1 mg—you will put it in?"

"Yes!" I say, glad because now Sheila won't have to wait for the fellow to enter the order into the computer himself. I head down the hallway to the locked narcotics room, where I punch in the code, then key in my individual password to our Pyxis machine: the multi-drawer device that dispenses opioids and other pain medications. Rushing back, I stop and take the time to type the drug order into the computer. Paperwork delayed can end up forgotten and this is a narc. I need to do it right so it doesn't look like I'm stealing drugs. I record that an MD ordered the drug and that Sheila got the correct dose on time.

Done, I grab the plastic vial that contains the Dilaudid and twist off the top. Next I slide out the glass vial of drug and flip off the plastic cover. I tear open an alcohol wipe and smear it across the top of the vial, then stick in a needled syringe, turn the vial upside down, and pull out the ordered dose of Dilaudid: 1 mg/1 ml. Good. Then I slide the plastic off one of my 10 ml syringes of saline, enjoying the satisfying "pop" sound it makes, and inject it into the 1 ml of narcotic. Most patients aren't chronic users of opioids and they don't like the heady, dizzy feeling that comes from getting the drug straight, so I always dilute it in saline for their comfort.

In the room I notice that the fellow is already gone. Maybe he couldn't get Sheila to talk much. She seemed in so much pain. I unwrap another syringe of saline and rub alcohol over the lowest hub—or opening—on Sheila's IV tubing. She's getting the blood thinner Argatroban and it's safer not to push the Dilaudid through that drug, so I pause her pump, pinch the tubing above the Y-site, and push in 10 ml of normal saline to clear Argatroban out of the stretch of IV line immediately below the hub. Then I clean the connector with alcohol again and push in the diluted Dilaudid. After that I use another alcohol wipe and push in another 10 ml syringe of saline. Finally I release the tubing, smooth it out, and restart the pump. Sheila's Argatroban returns to its slow drip.

I lower my face to where her head is below the blankets. "That should work pretty quickly," I tell her. "So let me know if it doesn't."

I pull back just a little of the blanket and put the stethoscope on her back so I can listen to her lungs. "I'm giving you a little bit of a check," I tell her, measuring her heart rate at her wrist. I look at her feet for any swelling (which is a way to evaluate kidney and heart function), then cover her back up. I need to listen to her gut, but don't want to ask her to move until the Dilaudid's had time to work.

"I'll be back," I tell her, making a mental note to remember.

I don't linger. This is the part of the day when it's easiest to get behind. I'll check these systems on every patient, plus verify the change-the-date sticker on the IV tubing and check dates on the dressings that cover central lines. We want to keep patients from getting infections in the hospital, and that's why I'm obsessive about Purell and wearing gloves and always using alcohol wipes for IVs, too.

I gather together Mr. Hampton's morning pills and go into his room. He's lying in bed blinking himself awake, trying to rise to a sitting position, but he can't quite do it.

"Hi! I'm Theresa, your nurse today. I've got your morning pills," I tell him, holding up the individual pill packets with my right hand.

He bobs his head, sort of like a nod. "Do you want to sit up in bed?" I ask him. "I can help you."

He shakes his head: no. "Want to get some more sleep?" He nods again. I guess he decided that sitting up was too much effort.

"OK, let me just get in a listen," I tell him. I don't hear anything obvious in his lungs and the chart isn't clear about why he needs oxygen, just that he does. I hope he sounds all right. In the interests of infection control every patient gets his own disposable stethoscope and they don't work too well. We call them Fisher-Price stethoscopes. Not only are they bright yellow and hard plastic, making them look like a toy from a child's doctor kit, the sound quality is also similar.

I go through the rest of my routine, evaluating his heartbeat, belly, and feet. Then I check his IV line, a Peripherally Inserted Central Catheter or PICC, in his left upper arm, by rubbing alcohol pads on the end of each his two lumens, then attaching a 10 ml syringe of saline to each, injecting just a bit before I pull back on the stopper of the syringe, looking for the flash of blood that tells me the line is in the right place.

It's hard to imagine that the tip of a thin intravenous line could get dislodged inside a person's body, but it happens. I even had one patient who accidentally pulled his own PICC line out from his arm in the middle of the night without realizing it. Mr. Hampton's flushes smoothly and the flash of blood comes with little effort from me. I'll need to see that blood in the line immediately before he gets the Rituxan so it's efficient to verify that right now at least the line is working fine.

As force from the syringe makes blood swirl into the saline I stop and watch it billow like silk. Red. Beautiful. I never gave blood too much thought before I took this job, but now I revere it. Blood is the liquid of life. Red cells give oxygen, platelets form clots, and white cells protect us from infection. Without healthy blood humans cannot live. Seems obvious, I know, but working with cancer patients has made me unexpectedly respectful of this life force. I quickly take Mr. Hampton's pills out of their individual packages and leave them by the side of his bed in a pill cup. I'm not supposed to do that, but he's fallen back asleep already and I'm not sure I can get him awake enough to swallow them. In school they call this nursing judgment, just like my decision to wait to listen to Sheila's belly. At this moment neither of these things seems crucial. Of course, later either one might turn out to be.

I've got time, so I document on Mr. Hampton now. Nurses

used to "chart by exception"; we would note anything going on with the patient that deviated from normal and assume the rest was OK. Fear of lawsuits, combined with electronic health systems loaded with regulatory bells and whistles, has made charting more and more about recording everything possible about the patient, whether abnormal or not. Do the lungs sound clear? That's normal—chart it. Is the patient urinating? Normal—chart it. Having bowel movements? Chart that, but also specify the consistency, color, and frequency. Is the pulse steady and regular? That's normal, too, so make sure to chart it. Is the patient in pain? Pain gets charted if it's present or absent, even though lack of pain is also normal.

My concern is that over time charting has become a simulacrum of good care, rather than a record of it. A simple example: hospitals worry tremendously about patients falling down since falls can lead to regulatory hand slaps, additional costs of care that may not be reimbursed, and lawsuits, as well as, most important of all, patients getting hurt. The managerial response to this risk is to require more charting on whether a patient could fall. Every shift, I complete a full fall assessment on every patient, noting age, whether he's on narcotics, if he's incontinent and unsteady on his feet, and if there have been falls recently. The electronic health record then gives the patient a fall risk ranking of low, medium, or high. Each level of risk comes with a set of necessary precautions and I have to chart which ones I've done. Ideally I would do all of them.

The recommended safeguards are all excellent: make sure the call light is nearby, check on all high-risk patients regularly, tell them to ask for help before getting out of bed. Physicians such as Atul Gawande and Peter Provonost persuasively argue that checklists in hospitals save lives. Their work focuses on procedures and protocols, not assessments, but I also agree that carefully analyzing a patient's risk of falling is probably a good idea. It needs to be quicker, though, because the irony right now is, the time I spend on the computer carefully documenting a patient's fall risk is time I could physically spend in the patient's room talking about how we can work together to keep him upright and on his feet. Designers of electronic charting systems don't seem to understand that checklists themselves are not the innovation, because checklists are not substitutes for care. The real innovation is having staff use lists to consistently create the safest and highest-quality clinical environment possible.

Mr. Hampton is a true fall risk. He's older, on oxygen, and appears confused. He's been asleep so far this shift, but he could wake up needing to go to the bathroom at any time, feel uncertain about where he is, get tangled up in his sheets or oxygen tubing, and fall simply getting out of bed.

Thinking of that I feel a sudden sense of urgency and go and knock softly on Mr. Hampton's door. He's asleep again and I step over to the bed and tap his shoulder.

He opens his eyes and I pick up the plastic urinal on the shelf next to his bed. "Mr. Hampton," I say quietly, holding up the urinal with a gloved hand so that he can see it. "Do you need to go to the bathroom?" He nods and I help him sit up in bed by sliding one arm behind his back. Then I disentangle his legs from his heap of covers until he can dangle them over the edge of the bed, ultimately resting his feet on the floor. He is very tall.

"Do you need my help?"

He shakes his head no and reaches out for the urinal. With his other hand he reaches under the edge of his hospital gown and prepares to urinate. I turn sideways so that my back is to him, but I keep my right hand on his shoulder to prop him up and so that I'll feel it if he starts to lean forward precipitously.

I hear the sound of a urine stream and then it stops. I wait a few seconds, then ask if he's done.

"Hunh," he says. It's the first sound I've heard him make! I turn around to face him, pleased that he's verbalizing something, and with my other gloved hand take the urinal from him and set it aside. I grab a wet wipe from the packet in his room and hand it to him. He takes it and slowly and carefully wipes both hands, afterward handing the used wipe to me.

I look at the urinal. He really needed to pee. I bend down to put myself at eye level with him. "Better?"

"Better," he says, almost as if he's talking to himself, but his voice is strong with none of the quaverings of old age. I look at him, wrinkling my eyebrows together as I adjust the two plastic prongs that send oxygen into his nose. Already he's trying to get back under the covers and I help him slide his legs in and fall back on the bed.

His eyes start to close. I use the pulse-oxygen machine to

check his oxygen saturation and heart rate. All normal. Guess he's tired, I think, frowning to myself. All this sleeping is somewhat unusual but, of course, he's also sick with lymphoma.

In his bathroom I empty the urinal, measuring the amount so that I can record it later. All fluid that goes into and out of a patient gets charted, too.

I've now helped to keep Mr. Hampton safe, but the scary thing is that patients will fall no matter what hospitals do. They fall because they lunge for cell phones. They fall because their blood pressure drops too quickly too soon after they stand up. They fall because cancer is clouding their brain and messing with their cerebellum. They fall because they don't want to ask for help in the bathroom.

Humans are bipeds—it's easy for us to fall. My husband and I have both had bad falls walking the dog in sketchy weather. I would like to be encouraged to physically *observe* my patients rather than simply record that I *have* observed them. Today at least I documented that I kept Mr. Hampton safe from falling and I also had time to actually do it.

Suddenly I remember. I have to listen to Sheila's bowel sounds and I don't want to forget. Is this the small something I might easily neglect that could make all the difference for Sheila, similar to the many small but vital steps in the clotting cascade? Watching Mr. Hampton as he falls back asleep, head nested in the pillow, I think it through. Oh, that's right, I wanted to spare her pain. To have listened right then, when I was in the room, was the correct clinical choice, but it was not the best choice for Sheila overall. No harm, no foul, though; I can fix this.

I decide to hurry into Sheila's room, check her abdomen and see if the Dilaudid is working, then give Dorothy her pills. Except Dorothy's call light comes on and I hear it chime. Rock and a hard place. I'll see what Dorothy needs; I've already gathered her morning meds. I'll review them with her quickly, then see Sheila, and come back to Dorothy's room later for a chat.

I saved Dorothy for last because she always enjoys talking and she's made her hospital room as much like home as possible, so it's nice to go in there. Her glass candy dish is on the bedside table, she's covered one wall with taped-up family photos, and a card table in the corner offers visitors a perpetually half-finished jigsaw puzzle. A thick, purple comforter overlies the bed and Dorothy herself always wears loose gray sweat pants, pastel sweatshirts, and a series of floppy caps that disguise her lack of hair.

I go in, say hi, reach behind the bed to turn off the call bell. Dorothy looks preoccupied and I'm guessing she wants to know what her neutrophil count is, to know if she can go home. But she surprises me.

"Do you have my Prilosec?" she asks, her voice high, tremulous.

"Sure. It's right here," I say, tearing off the paper wrapper and dropping the pill into the plastic cup I've brought into the room.

"I need that Prilosec!" she says, and she has tears in her eyes.

"Breakfast will be here soon and I get such horrible indigestion." She shakes her bald head and her pink and white knit cap shakes with it. "Every day I ask to have my Prilosec earlier and I never get it when I want it."

I've never seen her like this. I wonder selfishly what happened to my sweet, motherly patient. And then, because I want to be kind and feel effective, I make a promise that most likely I cannot keep.

"I'll fix it for you, Dorothy," I tell her.

There are certain drugs that have to be given on time—insulin, chemotherapy, opioids for pain—but Prilosec, a drug that prevents heartburn, doesn't qualify for that list. I've never had a patient feel strongly about it.

"I'm awake at six a.m. and I could get my Prilosec anytime after that. It's already past eight right now." Her voice cracks—she's very upset about the Prilosec.

"I'll fix it for you," I say again, pained by her high, strained voice. I want to help her, but honestly, I can't guarantee Dorothy will get her Prilosec any sooner than she did today. It's scheduled for 7:30 and pills are rarely given earlier since most patients are asleep and there's typically no urgency. We're treating cancer here; no one worries about Prilosec . . . except for Dorothy.

I take her other pills out of their wrappers, announcing the name of each one as I go: voriconazole, Acyclovir, ciprofloxacin. I drop them into the pill cup and the light blue, pink, yellow, and white pills mix together like Easter eggs in a basket.

I do all my checks, which she just tolerates because she's

annoyed, and I ask the usual questions: "Besides the heart-burn, any other issues with eating? Nausea, vomiting, diarrhea, constipation?"

She shakes her head. I take out alcohol wipes and pop some saline flushes out of their wrappers, checking each lumen of her central line while she obligingly pulls down the upper right edge of her shirt to show me the dressing where the line goes in just below her right clavicle.

"Your line's working great," I murmur, satisfied with the flash of blood I see in all three lines.

Now I bend toward her, looking her right in the eye. Her fleshy face interrupted with a hard frown, she gives me a firm look. I couldn't have known about the Prilosec, but I feel I should have.

"I will try to make sure you get your Prilosec earlier, Dorothy," I tell her, gently shaking the cup of pills so that they rattle—a reminder to her to take them even though she knows the routine after being in the hospital for almost six weeks.

She nods, still irritated, and reaches for the pill cup, her water at the bedside.

"I'll be back." I give her a small frown, hoping it conveys empathy with her frustration. She's busy swallowing her pills and doesn't notice, but her shoulders have relaxed.

On my way out the door I grab a couple of Hershey's kisses from the candy bowl and eat them in the hallway without much noticing the taste. Breakfast?

Dorothy had AML—acute myelogenous leukemia—the

deadliest and most pernicious of the adult leukemias. The initial treatment requires an extended hospital stay and that's what she's mostly done with. In the first week the patient receives a seven-day blast of chemotherapy. The next five weeks are spent recovering from the chemo's side effects: mouth sores, diarrhea, vomiting, and pancytopenia, or a severe reduction in the numbers of white blood cells, red cells, and platelets.

We draw blood every day to track the fall and rise of patients' blood counts and when needed we give transfusions of red cells to control anemia and platelets to reduce the risk of spontaneous bleeding. White cells, unfortunately, can't be transfused like blood or platelets and not too much can be done to make them grow back faster, so the patients get sick easily and fast when the white count, and especially the neutrophil count, is at the nadir or low point, which is typically zero. Having a fast-moving infection raging through a body with very few defenses of its own is dangerous, and a large part of why AML patients like Dorothy usually stay in the hospital for so long. We nurses keep an eye on them—checking temperature, heart rate, blood pressure, and oxygen level every four hours—so that if there is a problem we can respond right away.

Truth is, having heartburn be her biggest worry is a welcome change for Dorothy, though I wouldn't put it that way to her.

Sheila. I should see Sheila, but first I go to the computer on my medcart and reschedule Dorothy's Prilosec for 6:30 a.m. I attach a note in the computer about how important it is to give Dorothy the drug at that time. Maybe it will work for the day or two before she gets discharged.

Now Sheila— "Hey, Democrat," I hear, and turn around, half-smiling, shaking my head. It's Dorothy's rounding team and the attending physician is giving me a hard time. "Are you actually doing some work?" He's on the youngish side, for an oncologist, but he teases me the way my older brother would. Except it's not quite brother and sister. He's flirting, mildly, and I'm flirting back.

"You're not just freeloading, right? Like most Democrats?" This is our usual joke, that our politics reveal me as lazy and him ridiculous. My being a Democrat and his being a Republican aside, our sparring is fun and I have no idea where his real political loyalties lie. He steps up to me now and puts his arm around my shoulders. He's my height, with short blond hair and thick cool-nerdy glasses. He smells vaguely of not-cheap cologne and I see a streak of razor burn above his crisp white collar. "Hey, Theresa," he says. "If I asked you to get me a cup of coffee would you do it?"

Hmmmm. This is a new wrinkle. When joking with attending physicians there's always a risk of crossing the line between teasing and impertinence, but this doc is skating very near the line between banter and insult. I can't let him get away with treating me like a servant, or a nurse from forty years ago. Plus, I feel on firm ground with this MD, who doesn't take himself too seriously.

"Sure," I say, "As long as I could bring it back here and pour it over your head."

We're being flirty, yes, but there's aggression here, too, some old-school doctor/nurse nonsense.

"Well, just as long as you bring it to me," he says, being boyishly charming. "That's what matters."

And then he drops his arm from around my shoulders and switches back to work mode. "OK," he says, "Dorothy Webb," and points at Lucy, the nurse practitioner, or NP, while we cluster around her in the hallway. Lucy's short and today has tamed her thick black hair with a bright red headband. She reviews Dorothy's history and updates the team—the attending physician, a clinical pharmacist, another NP, and a physician assistant, or PA—on Dorothy's status.

I've been discreetly charting my morning assessment on Dorothy on my medcart computer while listening to Lucy, and now I click to the screen with lab results to check if Dorothy's ANC—her absolute neutrophil count—has been posted by the lab. An ANC reliably above 500 indicates that Dorothy has enough of an immune system to go home and it's important to learn that number right now. Once again Sheila has to wait.

". . . ANC wasn't back yet . . . ," Lucy is saying, but after seeing that the lab has just posted the ANC. I interrupt.

"It's here!" I say, "And it's . . . Whoa, it's 850!"

"It's 850?" the attending says, "Well, let's go tell her!" He swings his arm holding his papers in an arc toward Dorothy's door, as if he's sweeping us all into the room. We happily follow en masse. Moments like this are why we're all here.

"Your ANC is 850!" the attending announces and Dorothy claps her hands in her bed. If she had heartburn this morning it seems to be OK now. Or maybe she's so excited about returning home that she doesn't care.

"So that means," the attending says, "that someone has to

do the neutrophil dance." He looks at me, "Theresa! Do the neutrophil dance."

Startled, I look around the room. I've heard of the neutrophil dance, but I thought it was a joke, hospital legend, not an actual thing that real people actually perform. Is the attending physician trying to make me look foolish?

Everyone's looking at me, including Dorothy, and I realize there are worse things than embarrassing myself for her sake, a lot worse. Recalling movements from ballet classes of years past I wave my arms around above my head, more or less fluidly, and shimmy my hips, feeling pretty ridiculous, but the whole room cheers, and Dorothy once again claps her hands like a child. This is the Dorothy I'm used to—pleasant and forbearing. I'm glad this news came when it did; once Dorothy is home she can take her Prilosec whenever she wants.

She looks at me and laughs and I smile back.

"So you get to go home," the attending says. "Today, if you like." He gets a sly look on his face, "Or you can stay another day if you'd rather."

"Oh, no," she answers back, her knit cap shaking emphatically "Today is just fine. I'll call my husband and start packing."

A chuckle goes around the room. The attending points at her now, leaning his body forward. "Lucy and Theresa will get you out of here," he says, slicing his right palm across his left in a quick motion. "Lickety-split."

"Well, not too fast. My husband has to get here."

"Don't worry, Dorothy," I reassure her, "Nothing happens too fast in the hospital if it involves paperwork."

"Oh, that's right. Well, I'll get started anyway," she says.

"As soon as you all leave." We laugh again and then troop out and that's it, an ordinary day shot through with the crystalline illumination of earned success, a gem-like moment. There's paperwork to do and it will all take longer than it should, but I'm contented. Dorothy's month and a half on the floor accomplished what we hoped, and she is finally going home.

Her team moves down the hall to its next patient, and I see the owlish intern for Mr. Hampton trailing behind his own attending physician and the rest of that group, heading in the opposite direction up the hall. Damn! I missed rounds on Mr. Hampton while I was in with Dorothy and her team. I wish the medical staff would call the nurses for rounds, include us, but they never do, and because I wasn't part of rounds I lost my chance to understand why the benefits of giving Mr. Hampton Rituxan are worth the possible risks. The intern looks preoccupied; he's probably already thinking about his next case. I won't be able to check in with him until later.

The woman from dietary shows up at my pod with her large warming cart full of trays. Breakfast is late today, but that's probably good for Dorothy's heartburn. The woman takes a tray in to Mr. Hampton, whom I'm guessing won't eat it. Sheila probably won't either. It's odd how little attention I pay to what my patients eat. I notice *if* they eat and if they don't, especially if that lasts for several days, but the food itself barely registers. If I think about it I know why that is, too. I'm not responsible for the food, so I wall it off in my mind, make sure it never goes on my mental list. What I do notice is patients feeling bad about, in their words, wasting food, because either cancer, or chemo has taken away their appetite. It's amazing how deep those messages about eating go. I tell them they've got cancer, so they have enough on their plate and don't need to fret about whatever they don't eat. Now I realize I'm comforting them with a metaphor that is itself about food.

Sheila's medical team gets to my pod—all the rounding groups are coming at almost the same time, unfortunately. I don't recognize anyone except for Yong Sun, the fellow, who gave me the Dilaudid order this morning. He gives me a discreet wave as the intern, a very tall woman with straight brown hair she wears long and parted in the middle, says "Sheila Field" and starts to talk in that breathless way most interns have, trying to get all the words out before being interrupted.

This is how rounds work. The person on the team with real-time responsibility for the patient that particular day—an intern, resident, NP, or PA—verbally delivers the relevant clinical information about that patient to the entire rounding team. Called "presenting the patient," the idea is that everyone on the team learns while listening. The attending physician responds by grilling the presenter into silence, or more ideally, by asking the presenter questions designed to make him or her think. A good attending physician instructs the entire team by explaining his or her thought process and treatment decisions, but the behavior and teaching style of all of them vary widely, as might be expected.

The residents—also called "house staff"—switch their clinical placement every month and the attendings sometimes change even more frequently than that, so the composition of the teams is always in flux. The NPs and PAs make up a permanent team, without interns or residents. The fellow, who stands in the hierarchy between the residents, NPs, PAs, and the attendings, can throw a life preserver or a wrench into the works. Most everyone has good intentions, but chemistry can be bad between members of the team, speaking styles can vary, even expectations won't always be the same.

I don't know Sheila's attending well. Balding, with the beginning of middle-aged spread and his lab coat pockets drooping from too many stuffed-in papers, he listens distractedly. I read his name, Nicholas Martin, on the tag clipped to his white coat.

"Came in from an outside hospital," the intern says, "... coagulation disorder ... abdominal pain."

I stand in their circle, concentrating. Dr. Martin grimaces and says, to no one in particular, "I'm an oncologist, not a hematologist." He's complaining that he's trained to treat cancer patients, not people with unusual clotting problems. Sheila doesn't have cancer, but her disease is rare enough that despite being a teaching hospital we don't have an MD onsite 24/7 who specializes in her particular illness. An oncologist who's also trained in hematology is the best we can do, but throw in Sheila's mysterious abdominal pain and Dr. Martin is out of his element clinically, which annoys him, probably because it makes him insecure. He may feel he's not expert enough to care for her.

Regardless, the interns and resident look at him expectantly. They may get his point—that he's not the ideal physician for Sheila—but they have their own pressures to contend with.

They're on the floor to learn how to be doctors and the attending is there to teach them. He will not help them juggle their many responsibilities by doing some of the day-to-day work that keeps them busy, and they will be equally as abstemious with their empathy for the clinical predicament in which he finds himself. It's the way the hierarchy works.

"Could be HIT" he says, half to himself. He's talking about heparin-induced thrombocytopenia. People pronounce HIT like the word "hit," but I always think it should be "H-I-T" because that makes it sound a lot more serious. "Hit" is kids squabbling, but H-I-T, like HIV, is a disease.

Doctors like to tell stories about the rare but tragic case they will always remember, but we nurses have our stories, too, and mine involves a patient with HIT. I met this man when I was a nursing student. He'd come into the hospital for what was supposed to be a routine cardiac test and ended up with a new heart, the lower half of his right leg amputated, and toes dying on his still-intact left foot. An emergency heart transplant had saved his life after a routine cardiac procedure went very wrong, but the heparin he received to prevent blood clots after the open-heart surgery gave him HIT: a rare but very serious allergic reaction to the drug. Heparin is supposed to extend the clotting time of blood, but with HIT the reverse happens and blood clots when it shouldn't.

For this patient clots formed in both of his legs, leading to massive tissue death and the amputation, and he was facing the possible loss of his left foot, too. At one point he half woke up and wanted only to die. Then a few days later he really woke up and his wife was there, his sons. He changed his mind. What-ever it took he wanted to live as fully as he could.

That was the first time I really saw that our attempts at healing can do harm. Everything that happened to this patient fell into the range of rare-but-acknowledged-risk, and the guy was lucky he wasn't dead. His life was forever changed after receiving our "care." He would need anti-rejection medicines for his new heart and have to learn to walk all over again with a prosthesis in place of the leg he'd lost. Changing the bandages on his dying toes caused a shadow of pain to fall over his face, like the moon covering the sun during an eclipse.

Outside Sheila's room the intern suggests a few blood tests to run. I hope they show that Sheila does not have HIT. Dr. Martin nods. "Order a scan of her belly, too," he says. That's routine, a good idea, I think. They're getting ready to go into the room when the other intern gets a call on his cell phone. He looks startled as he relays the message, but his voice is steady. "Chardash, that patient on five north, is decompensating." A different patient somewhere else in the hospital, maybe a cancer patient we didn't have room for on one of the oncology floors, is spiraling down.

"Well, then we need to go there," the attending says. "We'll come back here. But get everything we talked about started," he says, with a flick of his wrist to indicate that the tall, thin intern should enter her orders.

"Tell me more about Chardash," I hear him say as the team quickly moves up the hall to get to the fifth floor.

The intern hurries up to the nurses' station to put in the orders she suggested on rounds and I'm left alone and disappointed and, I realize as my stomach growls, hungry. I grab two packs of Saltines from the small patient kitchen across the hall and eat the plain crackers meditatively while standing in front of my medcart re-reading the notes I have on Sheila. It seems like no one on the team was very interested in figuring out what was up with her. They probably just didn't have the time, but this is when I miss being in a university, a place where people could stand around and talk exhaustively about all sorts of arcane concerns for hours. I wanted a mini-seminar on antiphospholipid antibody syndrome, a fuller explanation of why Sheila had to come here at three in the morning, but instead I got the silence left in the wake of an emergency.

"Hey, can you help me with a transfer? My patient came back pretty sedated; I'm gonna need some help moving him." It's Susie again.

I swallow the last bite of Saltine. Mr. Hampton needs to take his pills and Sheila's belly has not been listened to by me, but Susie needs help now. The escorts who move patients to and from different places in the hospital are blamed if they fall behind schedule. Patients dislike waiting on the hard carriers since their beds are a lot more comfortable. And Susie's new—she's learning about nurses having each other's backs, or not.

"Let's go." I tell her.

"You sure?"

"I've only got three patients."

"Three? You're so lucky. My four are keeping me jumping."
We're walking down the hallway, back to her pod.

"It's a busy time on the floor," I tell her.

In the room Randy, another fairly new nurse, is also waiting. The guys often get called in for transfers and Randy was an
EMT so he's good at moving people.

"I'll come on the other side of the bed with you, Susie," he
says, "Theresa, you grab the feet."

We take our positions. The patient doesn't look that heavy,
but bodies can be deceiving.

"Can you get that IV line up and out of the way?" I gesture
at the escort, who's ready to push from her side of the carrier.
She lifts up the plastic tubing and lays it on the patient's chest.

"He's too out of it to help," Susie says. "So, one, two, three!"
We each pick up our section of the patient, slide it to the right,
and lay it down with a gentle thud. It was a smooth transfer. The
patient briefly opens his eyes, then closes them again.

"Very nice!" Randy says. He looks at the patient, who seems
sound asleep. "Jeez, what'd they give him down there?"

Susie scrunches her eyes together, then remembers. "Conscious sedation, but he barely slept last night—he got platelets
and his pump kept beeping. He was really tired." Randy gives a
quick nod. That makes sense.

"You good in here?" I look at Susie and the escort while
sliding between the carrier and the bed to raise the bed rail up
and next to the patient. We don't want him falling out.

"Yup. Thanks!" Susie confirms.

"I'll get this carrier out of here," Randy offers, and pushes it into the hall, stripping off the dirty linens after he gets it there.

I see the patient's physical chart in his room. "I'll take this up to the nurses' station," I call out to Susie.

As I head up the hall I dial down my impatience about Sheila. She's getting a drug that will make her blood clot more slowly and we're drawing the appropriate labs and getting a scan of her belly. It's not dazzling clinical work, not the Sherlock Holmes of medicine in action, but then again most of modern health care doesn't consist of intense deduction followed by "Aha!" moments. Smart, hard-working people gather data, ponder for however long they've got, and then act. Time is always of the essence.

Speaking of time, I look at my watch. How did it get to be 9:30 a.m. already? And I didn't call home. I used to make a point of always calling home in the morning before the kids left for school. I loved hearing their little soft voices, imagining the bustle of lunches being prepared, backpacks being loaded and zipped up. They usually didn't have much to say to me, but I wanted to let them know I was thinking about them. It seemed important.

Paradoxically, once I got more experience under my belt I stopped calling home in the morning. If I think about it I have to admit that not calling is actually easier. A call makes home, my actual home, too real and thinking too much about home might make me vulnerable in ways the job doesn't really accommodate. It's the patients who get to be emotional and unpredictable, not the staff, or at least that's the ideal. I need to be in control at work, so I don't call home unless I have to. I stick the chart for Susie's patient back in the circular rack and one of our social workers pulls it out immediately. "Is he your patient?" she asks, hopefully.

"No—Susie, down the hall," I point. Many hands make light work and that's good, because the sickest patients need a team of people to look after them.

Sheila's thin intern is talking on the phone and I overhear her. "Chardash was fine? Oh, that's good. Just a problem with his oxygen?" Sheila continues to wait for a full consideration of her health status, but I feel relieved that Chardash, a patient I've never heard of and know nothing about, has been rescued from whatever trouble seemed to be heading his way.

CHAPTER 4

Worries

*R*apid response team" comes over the PA sys-
tem and I wait, holding my breath, to find out where. "*Medical
Oncology.*"

Shit! Our floor? Which room? "It's here! It's Mr. King!" I
hear Nora. She's in the pod next to mine.

I walk back to her, fast, and see Susie coming down the hall,
fast, too, with Randy behind her. Nora has already pulled the
crash cart into the room and I see, quickly, Mr. King, a patient
most of us have known for over two years, lying in bed not moving with a thin stream of blood running from his mouth down
his chin onto his chest.

My focus narrows to what's right in front of me: the portable defibrillator is on the bed next to Mr. King. I grab the
small plastic instrument we use to measure oxygen saturation
and stick his finger into it.

"What's his pulse-ox?" asks Nora.

"Waiting." The machine registers a horizontal line as it calculates Mr. King's oxygen level. "Seventy-five percent."

"I'm cracking the cart, getting out a non-rebreather." That's Randy.

I hear Susie say, "What happened to him?" as I wrap the blood pressure cuff around his arm and start the machine so we can get his pressure.

Nora says, "I dunno. I walked in and found him like this. Here—you can record." She shoves a clipboard at Susie. "Write down everything that happens on this form."

Susie's eyes widen, but she takes the clipboard and clicks her pen open.

Suddenly the room floods with people: an ICU doc, nurses from the ICU, a respiratory therapist, an anesthesiologist. The code team has arrived.

This intensivist, Matt, is a friend. Despite not being any older than I am he's world-weary, but also whip smart with a well of compassion hidden beneath his hard edge. He stands by the opposite side of the bed, across from me, and our eyes briefly meet. Then he raises his voice above the loud buzz in the room. "What's up with this patient? Who's the nurse?"

Nora's good in codes. She rolls the information out like she'd memorized it. "Day one hundred–plus of a mud transplant, patient has GVH of the lungs and a fungal pneumonia, with increasing needs for oxygen. Alert and oriented with occasional moments of confusion, bed-bound due to weakness. Walked in this morning and saw him . . . like that, non-responsive. O2 sats

75 percent, so we put him on a non-rebreather." She points to the breathing apparatus now covering Mr. King's nose and mouth.

"His sats now?"

"Eighty-eight percent on twelve liters." Twelve liters is the maximum amount of oxygen that device can give and 88 percent is far below normal, which hovers between ninety-five and one hundred percent.

"Heart rate?"

"Fifty," someone calls out as Matt flips through Mr. King's chart.

"Pressure?"

"One hundred over eighty," I say.

"Let's get some blood gases," he tells the respiratory therapist. "What's his pressure? And what's his platelet count?"

"One hundred over eighty," I say again, louder this time, but I'm not sure Matt hears me over the ICU nurse calling out, "We have a bed! He can go to A222."

Nora also calls out at the same time, "Platelets are ten—he's refractory. No HLAs available." With a platelet count of ten, people can bleed spontaneously, and although we've been transfusing him regularly, his platelet count barely rises each time. (HLAs are platelets matched to Mr. King's blood, but we don't have any on hand. They can be hard to get.)

"Do I get to hear a blood pressure or not?" Matt demands.

I look at him and raise my voice. "It's one hundred over eighty," I say very loudly and he nods to himself. "OK, we'll take that bed. Pack him up and move him out. He's stable enough to transfer—we'll intubate him downstairs if we need to."

"Can we take him down in your bed?" the ICU nurse asks Nora. "We've got time—we can do it for you."

"You'll return our defibrillator? And the bed?"

"Uh . . . no. But you'll have to bring down his meds and give report. You can take them back with you then."

I have a sick taste in my mouth. Mr. King was my patient when he was first diagnosed over two years ago. He's gone up and down, but I thought he was in an up-phase. I haven't taken care of him for a while, though, so he must have gotten worse without my hearing about it. Having blood drip from his mouth and pool on his chest is unsettling since it suggests he didn't notice enough to spit or even turn his head to let it dribble out.

"Aspirated."

"He aspirated." It's a low murmur, passed person to person. Some of the blood from Mr. King's mouth went down the wrong tube, into his lungs.

"Has anyone called Opal?" I say. His wife. She's tough and resilient, but not prepared for this turn of events, at least not the last time I talked to her.

"I called her," says the nurse practitioner who's permanently on the stem cell transplant team. Mr. King is one of their patients. "She can't come right away, but as soon as possible." They live more than an hour's drive away and he's been in and out of the hospital for two years. God knows how she's keeping the rest of her life going in between times.

Nora, Randy, and the ICU nurses gather Mr. King's things—framed pictures, extra pairs of pajamas—and put them in some of our "patient-belonging bags." He'll have a lot less room in the ICU. Opal will have to take some of it home, I guess.

Matt has signed off on the rapid-response sheet that Susie filled out and starts to walk back up the hall when I flag him down. I lean in closer to him and keep my voice low. "What do you think his chances are?"

"Slim to none," he says, like he's swearing, and I hear in his voice that note of concern masked by resignation that made me like him the first time we met.

"That bad?"

He grabs my arm. "Theresa, we're all gonna die."

"Right, I know. But I like him," I say, trying not to sound childish.

"If you really like him, then wish for the family to put him on hospice so we don't have to keep all this up in the ICU."

"No chance that he'll make it?"

He stops and looks at me for a minute without speaking. We're about the same height and our eyes meet. "His lungs are junk, we can't stop him from bleeding, and he's got an opportunistic infection that's barely under control."

"I'd forgotten about the infection," I say in a low voice, mostly talking to myself.

"Wish for hospice," he tells me, firmly, and we both start walking again.

At my pod we wave good-bye to each other. "Thanks for looking on the bright side."

He gives me a pained smile, then, "That's what I'm here for."

The ICU nurses start to roll Mr. King down the hall. A housekeeper will clean the room, making it ready for a new patient. Nora will give report to the nurse in the ICU, just like the day-shift nurses all got report this morning, then come back upstairs and record everything that happened on the computer. Susie documented during the code, but that was on paper. Half an hour, forty-five minutes, and the emergency is over, except it feels like Mr. King took a piece of my heart with him, and he wasn't even my patient today.

I stand at my medcart and close my eyes. I try to mentally pack away Mr. King and the blood running down his chin while scanning my notes. Dorothy. Dorothy needs patient-belonging bags, too, especially since she's brought so many items from home into her room.

I go to the supply room and grab a bunch of them. Dorothy's going home, not to the ICU, I remind myself. Remembering that doesn't make me feel better about Mr. King, but it makes me less sad overall.

Back in her room, Dorothy's talking on her cell phone. "Well, now I don't know what time, if you can just help Dad get ready." It must be her adult daughter.

I hold up the bags and she gives me a half-smile and a loose finger wave with her right hand. She's put on lipstick and it gives color to her whole face. The beginning of her transition to home.

"Just tell Dad to get here as quick as he can." Trying not to interrupt, I put the belonging bags on her bed, wave back, and turn to the door.

"Wait!" She snaps her fingers. "No, not you!" she says sharply into the phone. Covering the receiver with her right hand and pointing at the candy dish, she says, "Take some chocolate. Today's my last day."

I pick up the glass lid, see the silver glint of Hershey's kisses, and pull them out from among the gold-wrapped Reese's and green and red Jolly Ranchers.

"Thank you," I mouth, dropping them into my pocket. My phone rings as I'm on my way out the door.

"It's radiology, CT scan. Can your patient Sheila Field come down now?"

CT: Computated Tomography—X-ray on steroids. I look at my watch. It's not even 10:00 a.m. "Sure. That was quick."

"We had a cancellation. Want me to put it in for transport?"

"If you have time, that's great. Thanks. I'll get her ready."

As I leave Dorothy's room she continues to talk on the phone, distractedly kneading the plastic bags I gave her. "Forget about that old carpet right now," I hear as I shut the door.

Now I will listen to Sheila's belly before she goes to CT. Sloppiness seems like a slippery slope, so being thorough, even if I'm late, is a form of mental discipline for me. I enter her room as quietly as possible. It's completely dark and she remains a lump under the blankets. I reach out for her shoulder and gently squeeze it. "Sheila? It's Theresa again. Did the Dilaudid help?"

The blanket goes up and down—a nod. I kneel so that my mouth is at the level of her buried ear. "Sheila, they've ordered a CT scan of your abdomen, to make sure everything is all right." The lump moves up and down again.

"Before you go to CT, I need to listen to your belly. Do you think you can roll onto your back?"

"Ungh," she says, with a grunt, and the lump rises and turns. The top edge of the blanket slips down and I see a pleasant-faced woman, in her late thirties, with thin reddish-blond hair that flows wispily away from a plump face. Her pale blue eyes are gentle, but lined, and her mouth has that frozen expression pain creates. The fingers holding onto the blanket are thick and there's a trustingness about her that makes her seem younger than she is, and vulnerable. She's all alone here, I think. I'll have to take care of her.

"This will be quick," I tell her.

I pick up the Fisher-Price stethoscope, rub alcohol on the ends, and stick them in my ears. I put the bell of the stethoscope down on the four quadrants of her abdomen—like two, five, seven, and ten on the face of a clock—and press lightly. Instead of the gurgling that's typical, I hear nothing, which is unexpected.

Why is Sheila's bowel quiet? It could be the cheap stethoscope. Or her having just woken up. Or my phone ringing right now as I listen, drowning out her abdominal burbles: "Escort. I'm on my way for Fields."

Or the rounding team returning, even though it's only Dr. Martin and the intern. "Now, Ms. Fields," the attending says peremptorily even though I'm bent over her with the stethoscope in my ears, "you've got a clotting disorder and your stomach hurts." Sheila nods, the fingers of both hands curled over the blanket's edge so that she looks like a child, trying to hide.

"We're giving you argatroban. We'll get a CT of your belly

and look at your blood work. It'll all get sorted out eventually. You should be home in a couple of days." He gives her a tight smile and she nods, but it's unclear how much she understands. I don't fully understand what's going on, so how could she?

He pulls back the blankets and pushes firmly on her belly. She gasps and her eyes open wide, then squeeze shut as she quickly pulls in her breath. "That's why we're getting the CT scan," he says, covering her back up with the blankets. "Anything else?" Dr. Martin looks questioningly at the intern, who shakes her head.

"They've already called her for CT," I say, wanting them to know what's happening.

"That's good," the attending says, but his tone doesn't change from that bland professionalism he used with Sheila. However, the intern gives me a weak smile. She and I are in this together.

I hear the electronic *ping-ping-ping* of my phone. "Transport. Here for Fields."

"I'm in the room—we're coming out." Dr. Martin signals for me to go out first. A little old-fashioned chivalry. Maybe he's not completely indifferent to the people around him. It could be he copes with clinical curve balls by withdrawing, or it could be he was taught to always let women go out doors first and that habit has never died.

The escort guy waits in the hall with an empty stretcher. He barely makes eye contact, but he's smooth with the carrier, like all of them. When I have to push a bed I'm an embarrassingly bad driver. The escorts make it look easy.

"Hey," I say, trying to be friendly. "You're here to take her to CT?"

"Fields," he says, half a question. I nod. "Can she walk?"

"She's in pain, but she should be able to walk." A piece of straight blond hair falls over the left side of his face. He's got a long-on-top haircut and that, combined with his funky thick-rimmed glasses make his burgundy uniform look almost cool. I can't recall ever, *ever*, having a real conversation with an escort. Never. Maybe that's why they often seem surly with us nurses.

It strikes me that my behavior with the escorts is not that different from the attending's behavior toward me. Maybe that means the attending, like me, is just trying to do his job as best he can. Or maybe it means we should all try a little harder to see each other as human beings.

I go back into the room and wake up Sheila. She's groggy but willing to move, if very slowly, and starts by sitting up in bed, grimacing.

"Can you stand up on your own or do you need my help?"

"I can do it." She breathes, starts to rise, then grips each of my arms as if they're chair rests. "Sorry." Her breath comes heavily.

"That's what I'm here for. You're fine."

She makes it all the way up. She's shorter than I am, heavy but not obese, and her hair is longer than I realized. It covers her shoulders like soft down.

She shuffles one foot forward. "You sure you can make it?" She nods, her mouth pulled tight, and shuffles the other foot forward. I feel for her and also feel fretful about how much time her slow walk is taking. Viewing time as the enemy has become a bad habit.

She reaches the stretcher and I see with relief that it's one of the newer ones that actually goes low enough for patients to sit down on like a normal chair. The escort and I help Sheila lie down on it. She looks more comfortable flat on her back, but the lines around her eyes stay tight.

"Hold on," I say, going back into her room to grab her pillow. "I'll be here when you get back."

The stretcher takes her away and I look at my watch: 10:10 a.m. I want to check in with my friend Beth about giving Mr. Hampton Rituxan. She's got more experience than I have and maybe she can help me feel less concerned about his ability to tolerate the drug, or have some advice about how best to monitor him when I give it. I remind myself that a rapid response team is always only a phone call away in an emergency and that whether Mr. Hampton lives or dies while getting his Rituxan is not solely on me, though I am the canary in his particular coal mine.

I would also love to get a coffee and something to eat, since my morning hunger is kicking in, but first Mr. Hampton needs to take the pills I left in his room. "Think you can take these now?" He's awake, but lying flat in bed, so I rattle the pill cup and try to look encouraging. He slowly moves his head up and down.

I raise the bed and help him situate himself so he can swallow safely. He needs my guidance to figure out where to move his torso, but not my strength to lift him.

I hand him water and he swallows the pills one by one with no trouble. "Great!" I say. "Want to lie back down?" He nods and I lower the bed, but something's off. He seems only vaguely aware of me and makes no sounds at all.

I peer at him, thinking, making the worry wrinkle, that vertical crease I get between my eyes. "I'll leave the room dark if that's what you want." But he's already curling back under the thin hospital blankets. Maybe he's just tired and doesn't feel like talking, but now I feel even more concerned about the Rituxan. It's an unpredictable drug. Most people who get it have no problems at all, others have mild reactions, some become quite ill, and a small percentage of those who become very ill die. It stands to reason that already being frail would translate into increased vulnerability to this hard-to-tolerate drug, but I don't know that for sure—I only have my worries.

Back out in the hallway I go to find Beth. Like me, Beth has twin daughters. Hers are all grown up, but she and I stand out among the mostly twenty-somethings on the floor and being moms of twins is a bond between us. Beth says our sick sense of humor is really what connects us. Like that time I asked her to witness me rinsing leftover narcotic down the sink: we have to give a reason for wasting opioids, but "patient died" is not one of the choices on the drug dispenser's computer menu, even though that was why I had a lot of morphine left over. Beth and I focused in on "patient refused" as a reason for wasting the narcotic, and the idea of it struck us both as so funny we laughed loud enough for people in the hall to hear us. The laughter was an acknowledgment of my grief, because I was actually quite sad about the patient's death and Beth knew that. I'll always remember the sadness of that shift, but because of Beth I'll remember the laughter, too.

Today, though, Beth doesn't seem up for humor. There's a grimness about her mouth that goes beyond the usual for work. She's preoccupied by something else.

"My daughter's flying to Kandahar today," she says, not looking away from her computer when I walk up.

"Your daughter, the one who's in the army?" Stupid question, but she nods.

"She left this morning, or whenever morning is over there." Now she looks at me. "I can't call. I can't email."

Hearing about a flight in a war zone, I picture brief clips from the movie *Black Hawk Down*: bullets, cornered soldiers yelling "RPG," the yellow dust of Somalia, and one stunning crash of a Black Hawk helicopter, propellers cutting sideways in slow motion as they hit hard-packed earth, black smoke funneling up and out of the wreck.

It will not be helpful to bring up any of this.

"Will you be able to work?"

"Well, being busy is good—it takes my mind off things."

That I understand. I don't call home because it feels too soft, too real, a threat to the game face I need to get through my day. For Beth, today, home is scarier than work.

She starts to add something else when my phone rings. "Sorry," I say to her and she turns back to her computer.

"You're getting a fourth patient and she'll be here soon." It's Nancy, the charge nurse, who is also one of our floor's two clinicians: she still works at the bedside, but also has set managerial tasks that take her away from patients. When Nancy's in charge her decisions tend to be whatever makes her day easiest. Some charge nurses will settle in the first admissions themselves to give the rest of us a break but others, like Nancy, never pick up patients.

"Admission for transplant; she got put on tomorrow's list by accident. You know her, it's Candace Moore."

Candace Moore. Shit. We *all* know Candace Moore. She's a PITA: Pain In The Ass. One Candace Moore can keep me as busy as two normal patients.

"You know I'm giving Rituxan later," I say.

"It's your turn to get a patient," she says. "The sheet's here at the nurse's station." I click off my phone. She's right that it is my turn, but Candace Moore . . . .

Candace brings her own supply of Clorox wipes to the hospital and has a rotating set of family and friends who help sanitize her room. She also writes down everything that happens and reads back over her notes with the intensity of an IRS agent studying tax returns, searching for damning discrepancies. Of course, with the very real danger of hospital-acquired infections and the large number of mistakes made in hospitals every year, I understand her obsessiveness. The problem is, she doesn't trust any of us. She wants our care but deep down, she's convinced we're here to hurt her, accidentally, or maybe even with malice, so she vacillates between aggressive suspicion and perky ingratiation. She lures all of us in with what looks like friendliness, only to turn against us when something, anything, triggers her paranoia. Being her nurse is the worst kind of no-win situation, which, if I'm honest, may be exactly how she feels about being a patient.

Early forties, Candace is youthful-looking, athletic and strong, but none of that matters much. She's coming in for an autologous transplant—an intravenous infusion of her own (cancer-free) cells—unlike an allogeneic transplant, in which a patient receives cells from someone else, called a "donor." Autologous transplants, or "autos," pose much less risk than allogeneic transplants, or "allos." The outcomes are also generally good for people with Candace's type of cancer, so objectively she has much less reason for anxiety than many of our other patients.

"An admission," I tell Beth, hanging up the phone. "I gotta go. Keep me posted," I say, sounding banal, but Beth waves as I walk away. At least I didn't complain about Candace; I also didn't get to ask her about Mr. Hampton. There's time, though.

At the nurse's station I pick up the patient printout the charge nurse left for me. "Candace Moore," the secretary says in a teasing voice, "Oh, T., you're gonna need some extra love today."

I frown. "Yes, well . . ."

The secretary laughs, then lowers her voice to a stage whisper. "Maybe she'll get here late. We can only hope."

Back at my medcart I'm wondering what time Candace will arrive, when *ping-ping-ping* my phone rings again.

"Medical Oncology. Theresa."

"Do you have Fields? This is radiology. What's she here for?"

His tone is urgent, his voice strained, and it throws me a little because I don't understand. I fall back on what I know: "She's got antiphospholipid antibody syndrome, we've started her on an Argatroban drip—"

"There's a lot of free air in her abdomen," he insists, cutting me off. We're back to her belly again. I'm not understanding. "That's a classic sign of a perforation."

A perf? Sheila's got a perf? No way—she's here with a clotting problem. A perforation is an emergency; she's got a hole in her gut that's leaking bowel contents into her abdomen. I can't comprehend what he's saying or connect with the urgency in his voice because Sheila is my "interesting medical" patient. My expectation is that we will manage her blood-clotting problem by monitoring laboratory values, making careful observations, and finding the right combination of drugs to control her disease. A perf is a surgical problem, as in only a scalpel can heal her, if even then.

Surgeons and nurses who work in OR inhabit a different world in the hospital from us medical folk. We work on floors with drugs; they use scalpels in sterile, well-lit rooms. We collect data and consider, while they cut out patients' problems with alacrity and skill.

There's an old joke about physicians going duck-hunting. The medical doc sees a bird flying in the sky and says, "It looks like a duck, and flies like a duck, and quacks like a duck, so therefore it must be a duck." He takes so long to determine that the duck is indeed a duck that it's flown away by the time he's ready to aim. Another bird flies into the sky and a different

MD, this time a surgeon, takes out his gun and shoots the bird repeatedly. It falls to earth with a thud and he walks over to look at it. "Yup," the surgeon says, "that's a duck."

We don't usually have surgical patients up here on the heme/ onc floor—we collect data and consider while they cut—but today it seems like I will. Absorbing this diagnosis is like moving a train through switches to get it on the right track. Sheila has a clotting problem, not a perf. But she has a perf, too. Click, click, click—my brain tries to adjust.

"Can you call the resident?" the radiologist asks, and his voice sounds very far away. I'm stunned, but now I get it. Sheila has a perforated, which is to say torn, intestine. There's a final click of the train track, then, "Yes, yes," I tell him. "I'll call." I hang up the phone.

This is bad. "A perf" is a phrase we learned to fear in nursing school because it is difficult to detect and deadly. I look on my paper for the intern's number and send a page with my phone number as the callback. I feel terrible that I had no inkling Sheila was so seriously hurt inside, but the truth is, diagnosing what's called an "acute abdomen" is complicated, and a scan is the only way to know for sure that a patient has perfed.

It's not the perforation itself that's so dangerous, though it will have to be surgically repaired; the gravest danger comes from the intestinal contents oozing from Sheila's GI tract into her open abdominal cavity. The insides of our bodies are sterile except for the parts open to the outside world, and while the human digestive tract is filled with bacteria that are essential for healthy digestion, those bacteria can become deadly if they proliferate in parts of our bodies that are supposed to be germ-free. In Sheila's warm, wet abdomen intestinal bacteria will multiply with little control, becoming an infection called peritonitis, which can become an even deadlier condition: sepsis.

Sepsis stimulates a catastrophic response from the immune system called SIRS for Systemic Inflammatory Response Syndrome. The acronym sounds polite but the reality of SIRS is not. At the late stages of sepsis, fluid from the blood stream moves into the body's tissues, leaving a reduced volume of blood in the arteries and veins. Due to this decrease in volume, the patient's blood pressure drops, and can keep dropping until there isn't enough pressure to send blood to every part of the body. When that happens, organs begin to shut down and die.

To picture what happens during the late stages of sepsis, imagine a garden hose with small holes placed throughout to turn it into a sprinkler. When a normal amount of water goes through the hose, the sprinkling effect is constant. If the flow decreases, the sprinkler effect becomes more erratic, and if the volume of water in the hose lessens even further, the sprinkler will turn into a leaky mess that waters only the strip of garden it rests on.

The tissues of our bodies are like that garden. Humans need constant watering with oxygenated blood—this is called perfusion—to keep our tissues healthy and alive. Human cells can become as parched for oxygen as carrots and zucchini in a garden become for lack of water, and if the flow of blood is too diminished the cells of our bodies will die, just like the vegetables in a drought-stricken garden.

Sepsis is a medical problem, but we can't treat only that—a surgeon must fix the hole in Sheila's gut to give her a chance of surviving this crisis. She's a medical patient on a medical oncology floor with a serious surgical problem and we have little experience with such cross-disciplinary cases in bone-marrow transplant. Sheila's perf puts me clinically out of my element, just like her attending physician, Dr. Martin, was out of his.

And then the guilt comes on full bore. Why didn't I see this coming? Why didn't I *know*? A good nurse has intuition; I believe that. I listened to Sheila's belly, but obviously I should have listened harder, better, thought more about what I was doing. My intellect was certainly piqued by antiphospholipid antibody syndrome. Was I not thinking about Sheila's abdominal pain because I was hoping that taking care of her would increase my knowledge of the clotting cascade and rare blood disorders? And is that why I didn't listen to her belly sooner?

Well, I'm learning a lot, but not what I hoped. Some years ago I had a different patient in the same room as Sheila, writhing and moaning with abdominal pain. Her husband was a yeller, one of those guys who's used to getting his way by being louder than everyone else. In the age of reimbursement based on patient satisfaction scores, nurses are discouraged from asking people to "please stop yelling because it makes it impossible for me to think."

I paged the oncology fellow because the husband insisted on what he called a "real doctor." The fellow came over, did a physical exam, and even though there was nothing indicating the need for a CT scan, there was a feeling of inevitability in the room. No matter what the fellow found, the wife would get that CT of her abdomen; and she did. There was no blockage of her intestine, not even a partial obstruction, and certainly no perforation. Cancer itself can cause extreme pain and pain medication was all she needed, though she did require a lot.

I realize now that the memory stayed with me as an example of sound and fury signifying nothing. I made the mistake of equating loudness of suffering, including the belligerent husband's, with clinical severity. His yelling intensified my concern for the wife, as it should have, but when we confirmed the wife's bowels were working fine, at least as far as the CT could show, I made that experience my baseline without thinking it through. In that situation there was lots of yelling and no perf. Therefore, a real perf would evince more moaning and writhing and even louder yelling.

A psychologist would call that a reaction formation: my outsize anxiety about a non-existent abdominal perforation led me to believe that if an actual perf occurs the patient will have a lot of pain and be very agitated. This, I now know, is wrong.

If there's one thing I should have learned in the hospital, it's how little control—of the good or the bad—we really have. Dorothy is cured and going home. Mr. Hampton is getting Rituxan and I am worried that it will hurt him more than help, or at the very least land him in intensive care. Candace is a hard patient to manage, but of course I want her transplant to go well. And now Sheila, my learning opportunity, turns out to be a slow-motion medical emergency.

My phone rings. "Medical Oncology. Theresa."

It's the intern. She's already heard from the anxious radiologist. "Stop the Argatroban," she tells me. She sounds scared or maybe, like me, she feels guilty for having no premonition about the perf. It's not rational that some of us who work in health care expect ourselves to be omniscient.

"If we stop the Argatroban now it will take several hours to clear her body. They can't operate until then." She hangs up.

I slide my phone back into my pocket and wonder who's going to tell Sheila this terrible news? Me? I would, but without any kind of plan in place I'd unnerve her without being able to list her options. I know very little about the surgery she will need.

My phone rings again. "Hey, it's Peter. Are you taking care of Sheila Fields?"

"Yes," I tell him. Click, another switch goes through; my mind is now mostly on track with Sheila's perf. Peter is Peter Coyne, an attending surgeon who is also a friend. The most common thing people say about Peter is, "I love Peter Coyne." He puts the lie to the common stereotype of surgeons as arrogant. He's sweet and a huge fan of bad puns and even worse jokes that I always laugh at despite myself. Whoever put in the consult for Peter to become Sheila's surgeon did a good thing for her.

We met a couple of years ago over the phone. He'd surgically placed a permanent intravenous line, a triple lumen Hickman catheter, in one of my patients and I needed to know if the line could be used. I was a new nurse and not as clued into the hospital hierarchy as I would eventually become. I called around to find out about my patient's IV line and someone told me to just page Dr. Coyne so I did.

My straightforward question, crisply delivered, "Is this newly-placed Hickman OK to use?" somehow devolved into a joke that made no sense but struck me as very funny.

"Well, I don't know," Peter said, "Are we placing Hickman catheters today or pumpkin catheters? If no one told you whether that line is safe to use I may just have to start handing out demerits."

The unexpectedness of his answer surprised me and I couldn't stop laughing. Then Peter got serious and told me the line was good and he would put an order to that effect in the computer.

"We'll be up soon, but I need to talk to her doctor," Peter tells me now. "Do you have the name?"

"I have the intern's name."

He laughs, but it's strained. "This isn't a case for the intern; I need to talk to the attending."

This is unusual. Attendings may talk to each other at meetings, or socially, I suppose, but on the floors they seem to only talk to each other through go-betweens such as interns or nurses or through scribbled notes that often don't even get read.

Attending to attending confirms my worries about Sheila. But Peter is on the case, so soon we will have a plan and it will be a good one. I think of the frustrated heme/onc attending, Dr. Martin. He was upset about having a patient with a blood disorder. Sheila's situation will only make him feel less capable of taking care of her.

"Nicholas Martin is the oncology attending."

"Oh, I know him," Peter says. There's something in his voice, not neutral, but I can't fix on it. "I'll call him." He hangs up.

I look down at the admission paper on my medcart. I need Candace Moore to take her time getting here because I'm short on patience, even though Sheila can't be operated on for hours because the Argatroban would make a complicated abdominal surgery even more dangerous than it already is. Because Argatroban slows clotting times, any cut would bleed much longer than usual and fixing a perf requires a large incision. Sheila's also overweight enough that she has thicker-than-normal layers of tissue to cut through for the surgery. The risks of excessive bleeding are obvious.

"You have no idea how much blood the human body holds," Matt, the ICU doctor from this morning's emergency, told me once, recalling what it was like to watch that precious fluid run out of a patient's body and cover the hospital floor when he had no ability to stop it.

But Sheila's stuck. The bacteria in her abdomen will multiply and spread while we wait for the Argatroban to clear her system. As time passes we swap one potential for death with another, but it's what we do here. The cutting edge of health care sometimes nestles just next to the razor's edge of survival. I check my watch. It's 11:00 a.m.: we'll have several hours of watch and wait.

I log into the computer, checking for any new orders on Dorothy, Mr. Hampton, or Sheila. All orders get recorded electronically and the computer is where newly placed orders pop up for nurses. While I think of it, I enter the verbal order the intern gave me to stop the Argatroban on Sheila and I write a note to myself to disconnect the drug once she's back on the floor. That should be soon.

But why wait? I call radiology and ask a nurse there to disconnect the Argatroban and ask her to tell Sheila there's been a change in the plan, which is true, even if my banal phrasing doesn't reflect how dire her situation is.

Ping-ping-ping. "Your admission is here!" the secretary says in her chirpy voice. Ugh. This timing is so bad. Not that I'm rushed right at this moment, but I'm worried about Sheila and preoccupied with my own useless feelings of guilt. Well, both of those will have to wait.

I quickly glance into the empty room between Mr. Hampton and Dorothy. Candace will start in on us right away if it's not, in her view, perfect. I repress my impatience as I see her push through the double doors toward me. She's pulling two designer suitcases behind her; she'll be here for at least a month. Her straight black hair is beautifully blown out. Is that a wig? I can never tell.

She smiles a big smile and I smile back, but I know the warmth she's offering probably won't last. Taking care of her usually feels like an emotional chess game.

"Candace. So it's really time for transplant."

She hugs me, giving my back a soft pat. She smells of citrus and expensive shampoo. "Well, first my dye study," she says and I squint at her because I don't understand.

"Dye study?"

"My Hickman's not working right," she says. She's had it

for several months now and they do malfunction. If we suspect a defect in the line, the patient goes to interventional radiology where they run dye through it while taking X-rays. It's a fairly precise way to show where the Hickman ends in the body and if each of the three lumens works correctly. "I told them I'm not having my transplant with this line until I have a dye study and that it's going to be today, right now."

I know I should just agree with her, but my curiosity gets the better of me. "What's wrong with it? Do you want me to flush it, check whether it's OK?" The lines are fairly simple mechanically and there are only a few things that can go wrong with them.

"No, I don't want you to check it; it's not working!" she bursts out, her voice almost shrill. "Would you want a transplant through an IV line that wasn't working? Or someone messing with it?"

"No," I say, shaking my head. Why did I ask her? "So that's today?"

"Yes, I'm just dropping my bags off and going down there."

"They're expecting you?"

"They'd better be," she says. I nod, smile again.

"Let me call transport. Since you're here as a patient, we'll want you to go down with an escort." I think for a minute, then explain hesitantly. "We'll need to send you with your chart, too, so there will probably be a little bit of a wait while we get that together." I try to sound pleasant, but firm, not like she's been here for five minutes and I'm already apologizing.

"Oh, that's fine," she says brightly, her mood once again

friendly, talkative. "No rush—my cousin's on her way in and we can clean the room while we wait." She holds up a grocery bag defiantly and through the thin plastic I see that it contains two large containers of Clorox wipes.

We go in the room and she puts one of her suitcases on the bed and tells me, without turning around, "I know you're busy—you just go do your work and I'll get settled in here."

In the hall, Nora, Mr. King's nurse, puts her hand up to her mouth and loudly whispers as she walks past, "Candace Moore."

"Good news travels fast, huh?" I say.

Breathe, I tell myself. *Just breathe.* Our bodies can't make energy without oxygen.

CHAPTER 5

Surgical Team C

Needing to clear my head I walk up to the nurses' station. When people ask why I left teaching English to become a nurse, it must be moments like this that puzzle them. Instead of being here at the hospital, concerned about madly proliferating bacteria and killer drugs, I could be discussing a novel with a group of interested college students. There's a lot more control in a classroom than in the hospital and no one's life was on the line as a result of my work in the Tufts University department of English.

I look up and there's Peter Coyne at the nurses' station, his white coat emphasizing the straightness with which he holds himself. He's tall and athletic-looking, with short-cut gray hair, and immediately he starts joking around with our secretary: "Someone said they tried to page me, but they didn't have a

Coyne for the phone." His smile is irresistible even though the pun is terrible. The secretary laughs and he keeps going: "To *Coyne* a phrase, did someone page me?" At the same time escort arrives back on the floor with Sheila.

Two of them have brought her, the blond guy from before and a short African-American woman with high cheekbones and long braided hair. They both have lives, hopes, and dreams, but the boundary between their world and mine is another that rarely gets crossed.

The stretcher is angled away so Sheila doesn't see me. I look in her direction quickly and see the Argatroban, unhooked on the IV pole, its tubing looped up neatly on one of the pole's metal hooks. The nurse in radiology hung a bag of normal saline in place of the Argatroban and I see that it's infusing—I'll check the orders and make sure the intern put that order in.

I should go over to Sheila and explain what's happening, but instead I gesture discreetly toward her room. I want the two escorts to get Sheila into bed without my help because I'd rather talk to her after I've checked in with Peter and have solid information to deliver.

The whole system should probably put more of a premium on giving patients disturbing news quickly. If it were me I would not want to discover that someone else had secret information about whether I might live or die and didn't tell me. But then again, I also wouldn't want them to frighten me with bad news if they weren't *sure*.

Peter keeps joking and I feel my impatience, so I interrupt him, "Let's go. I'm worried about my patient."

He stops joking and looks at me, suddenly earnest. "Does she need to be in the ICU?"

I think about it. "No. Her pressure's been good—she's stable." Since the bacteria multiplying in Sheila's belly will make her sicker over time and the overarching fear is sepsis, paying attention to her blood pressure is critical. Having Sheila's blood pressure remain normal or high is good right now. If she starts to drop—like the water pressure failing in the garden hose—we'll know she's getting sicker fast.

Peter and I head down the hall to Sheila's room. I'm ready to go in with him but the medical student who's been trailing us gestures at me in front of the computer in the hallway. He has a question.

These poor medical students. They worked so hard to get into med school and then in the hospital no one gives them the time of day, in part because they have no real purpose, at least on our floor. They're supposed to be learning and I'm sure they are, but as far as we nurses know they can't *do* anything. Plus, the white jackets they wear, deliberately shorter than the long white coats of the interns, residents, and attendings, make the male students resemble those little boys in old photographs wearing short pants.

I don't know why the medical student thinks it's my job to explain our software to him and I don't mind, usually, but his timing sucks. I squeeze my lips together, holding in frustration, then arrange my face to look neutrally helpful. Clueless now, he'll be a full-fledged doctor someday and I want him to see that nurses can be collegial.

He wants two small things explained: how to look up laboratory results and where to find the radiology report on Sheila. Geez, don't they teach the students anything before they start in the hospital? In a couple of years they'll be residents practicing medicine on real patients, but until then it's like no one even tells them where the bathrooms are.

This guy is nice despite his nervousness. Questions answered, he heads toward Sheila's room and I'm right behind him when my phone rings. It's Lucy, the nurse practitioner, wanting to update me on Dorothy's discharge. There will be dose adjustments in a few of her meds, so it's going to take a little longer.

"OK." I hang up and reach for Sheila's door when the phone rings again. "This is Trace Hampton. Richard Hampton's son." His voice is pleasant and direct and he asks me not to start the Rituxan until he can be there, around three in the afternoon. I look at my watch. It's 11:00 a.m. Considering I don't have orders yet that should be fine. "No problem," I tell him.

Then the phone rings again. It's Sheila's intern, the one with the long hair parted in the middle who smiled at me to show we were on the same team. "What's going on? No one's told me anything."

"The surgical service is already here," I tell her. "And I've stopped the Argatroban. Beyond that I have no information except we probably won't be moving her to the ICU."

"Can you call me when you find out anything?"

"Sure." I remember my question for her. "Did you order fluids?" I haven't had time to look it up on the computer yet.

"Yes. Normal saline at seventy-five."

"Great. I'll page you when I know what's up." I push the off button and see Peter and the medical student heading back up the hallway. I missed Peter's entire conversation with Sheila.

He turns around and flashes me that irresistibly friendly smile. "See ya later," he calls out, giving an exaggerated wave.

"What?!?" I say, playing along with what I think is a joke. It has to be a joke—how could he leave without filling me in? But my phone rings again so I can't quick-step after him to make sure.

"We have a Candace Moore down for a dye study and imaging today. It's not clear what exactly the problem is, though . . ."

It's interventional radiology and I don't have an answer for them beyond her telling me her line wasn't working. "Um."

"'Cause we just got two emergencies, so we're gonna have to push her back a few hours, OK? We'll call you when we're ready for her—it'll be a while." He hangs up.

I absolutely should go in to see Sheila, but first I run my eyes down my papers. Dorothy has a med due and I need to find out if Mr. Hampton is any more with-it than he was. I should also tell him about his son's phone call and that we won't start the Rituxan until at least three p.m. And now I have to tell Candace that her trip to IR has been delayed and hope she takes it well.

Prioritizing: The problem is, Dorothy will want to chat, and while I enjoy chatting with her I don't have time right now. I get out her pill and steel myself for a quick getaway only to discover that my planning was unnecessary. She's once again on the phone to her daughter (or maybe she never hung up?)

discussing her discharge. I set down the pill in its little plastic cup and wave. She waves back by wriggling her fingers in her usual way while talking. "Now when I get home we'll have to wash all the drapes. And maybe we should have the carpets cleaned. Also . . ." I leave. I can only imagine the domestic whirl-wind Dorothy is going to be after being away from her home for more than a month. As I head out the door she's saying, "No, of course I won't be doing the cleaning myself!" I smile. Her daughter will make sure Dorothy takes it easy, whether she wants to or not.

Mr. Hampton is sleeping again when I go into his room, but he's more alert when I wake him up than he was before. I give him the message from his son and he nods. He seems to know where he is, but his breathing is not easy.

Now to inform Candace about the delay. If my life were a play, this would be the moment of French farce—going in and out of adjoining rooms never knowing what I'm going to find on the other side.

I knock on her door and walk in. "Thank goodness," she says, raising her face to me, her eyes squinty with anger. "That shower curtain is moldy and look at this—look!" She holds out her hand, protected with a latex glove, and I glance down at it, seeing in her palm a quarter-sized ball of tangled hair and lint.

"That's, um . . ."

"Dirt! We found it behind the bed. *On the floor!*"

I swallow. We clean constantly in the hospital because residual dirt is never just mess. Methicillin-resistant Staphylo-coccus aureus (MRSA), Vancomycin-resistant enterococcus (VRE),

Clostridium difficile—these are the bacteria that live in hospitals and even sometimes in rooms that have been thoroughly scrubbed. A microscope might reveal Candace's dust bunny as a deadly disease vector. That is not a joke. She will be severely immuno-compromised after transplant, making her susceptible to infections that wouldn't ever trouble a healthy person.

I swallow again. Hospital administration recently laid off some housekeepers to save money and the ones left on the job now have too much to do. As with nursing and doctoring, mopping and wiping can only be speeded up so much before efficiency degenerates into missed spots.

"That's why *we're* cleaning the room," she says, and her cousin nods aggressively, keeping her back to me as she carefully rubs the windowsill with a Clorox wipe.

There's nothing to do but make things better from here on out. "You're right about the room."

"I know that!" she says, but her eyes are more relaxed. She's probably used to people treating her as though she's annoying rather than correct. Score one for empathy.

"You may not like this, either," I say, "but IR just called and they have to push back your dye study. They got two emergencies back to back."

"Oh, that's OK," she says, wiping down the stainless-steel bed rails. "Tell me when they're ready for me, but don't forget the new shower curtain! That shower curtain is disgusting!"

"She could die from that shower curtain," the cousin throws in.

"Right. New shower curtain." I slink out of the room without even checking to see if it really is moldy. It's a five-dollar shower curtain. After the hair-and-bacteria ball under the bed I'm not going to argue.

Out in the hallway I call maintenance before I forget. "OK," the guy says, and I hang up, relieved that for once I could tell someone about something needing to be fixed and they would agree to do it without my having to explain.

Ping-ping-ping my phone rings again and this time it's Peter calling me; he's back on the floor. I look at Sheila's door. I should go in, see how she's doing. But it's easier to ignore a closed door than a live person on the telephone. "I'm coming right now," I tell him, putting my phone in my pocket and walking to the nurses' station.

He sits in front of a computer surrounded by a flock of surgical interns and residents, bright in their long white coats. One is on the short side with red hair and freckles on his plump cheeks, another is tall with a long face. And then I see my real-life next-door neighbor, Akash Patel. Young, handsome, from an Indian family, he grew up in the South and now lives in the house adjacent to mine. Akash is very smart and very nice. His wife is sure he works too hard, which I think is a common feeling among doctors' spouses—women and men.

A surgical team encamping on our medical oncology floor in the middle of the day is unusual. Dot, the veteran nurse with a bottomless reservoir of common sense and a sly smoky laugh, sidles up next to me. "What's going on?" she whispers.

"My patient, Fields, has a perf."

"Oh shit," she says, scrunching up her face. "When?"

"They just found it on CT. She came in last night from an outside hospital."

"Are you OK?" This is a hospital question that asks about much more than it seems to: Is your patient stable or could she spiral down at anytime? How's the rest of your load? Are you calm or panicked at this emergency?

"Right now I'm good, but I've got Candace Moore."

"Oh . . . shit." Her great laugh comes low and deep.

"And I'm giving Rituxan later to a seventy-five-year-old on oxygen."

"Who thought up that assignment? Oh wait, let me guess." Her eyes slide over to the charge nurse.

"You got that right," I say.

"Hey," she says, serious now. "You can only do what you can do, and you know where to find me if you need help."

"Thanks," I squeeze her arm and turn back to the flock of surgeons.

"Hey," I say to Akash, who nods his head back at me. I jerk my thumb toward him and ask Peter, "Did you remember that he's my next-door neighbor?" Peter and I had talked about Akash before.

"Oh, that's right," he says, not taking his eyes off the computer screen.

"So, are you being nice to him?" I ask.

Peter looks up. The air feels electric. I may have crossed a line, just like Dorothy's attending did this morning when he teased me about getting him coffee. This line isn't doctor-nurse, though; it's resident-attending. Peter *is* nice, but at the moment he is also my neighbor's boss and it's not my place to pester him about that no matter how many bad jokes he makes with our secretary or how good my intentions.

He turns back to the computer screen unperturbed, though, and begins planning out loud. "Stopped the Argatroban around 10:00 a.m.—let's say 11:00 a.m. just to be safe; so we probably can't operate until five at the earliest depending on her clotting factors." He stops to think for a moment. "Have to call the on-cology attending, see if we can give her anything to speed that up. What's her pressure?"

"It's been high," I say while he scans the computer, "160 over 100. Though I haven't checked it for at least an hour."

Akash says, "That's fine. And better too high than too low," while the other residents nod.

"She'll have to see anesthesia," Peter continues. "They'll talk to her—for a really long time—plump her pillows, get her ready."

"Will they give her tea?" I ask, playing along with his joke.

Peter glances at me and says, "With cookies," then turns back to the computer screen.

Finally looking up from the computer screen, he announces, "I'm giving her to Akash. You'll be the resident in charge of her case."

This is excellent news for me. It's much easier to work with someone you know than someone you don't and even better if you know you like them.

Peter's pager buzzes and he pulls it off his waist, checks the number, and nimbly reaches for the phone next to the computer. Akash walks over to me. "What's her IV access?"

"She's got a twenty-two gauge in her left arm."

"Do you think it will hold?" He's asking me if her IV will stay functional. The non-permanent intravenous lines can go bad at any time, though they usually work well enough for at least a couple days.

I raise my hands in an "I don't know" gesture: "It's working."

"Fluids?"

"Normal saline at seventy-five."

"Let's increase that to one fifty. We want to keep her plenty hydrated."

I nod. "I'll put it in as a verbal."

He looks at his watch. "You'll be home late tonight," I say. "Tell Monique that it's all my fault."

He laughs, then asks me to write down his cell number. "Can you call me when she's on her way to the OR? It just makes it easier." He sounds apologetic and I'm surprised that he's asking me to call him directly rather than paging and waiting for a call back. That we carry phones, which have to be answered when they ring, whereas doctors have pagers that they can, at least briefly, ignore, sometimes feels unequal to me. But I also know that a page can be just as disruptive and annoying as a phone call. Docs aren't as immediately on the hook as we nurses are with our phones, but the pressure to *call back* ASAP must be fierce.

I spent a day shadowing in the emergency department when I was in nursing school. An elderly woman who'd fallen needed a hole drilled in her skull to relieve the pressure from a bleed in her brain.

A neurosurgery resident was called in to do the job and a more tired-looking human being I hadn't seen in a long time. His face was ashen and being unshaven only emphasized the lack of color on his cheeks. His scrub pants were too big and too long and his scrub top was so wrinkled it looked as though he'd slept in it.

He held the drill up to the back of the patient's head with a narrowing of his eyes, hoping focus would keep his hands steady. As the drill went in small pieces of bloody tissue and bone spattered out behind the unconscious patient.

His pager kept beeping. Every time it beeped he would stop the drill, put his right forearm up to his forehead, pick up the pager and look at the number, then go back to the drill until the pager beeped again.

I thought that if I were having a hole drilled in my head I would not want the person doing it to be constantly interrupted, or interrupted at all. I picked the pager up from where he'd left it on the stretcher and mimed that I would be responsible for it until he was done.

He shifted his eyes over to me quickly and gave one shallow nod. Then he returned to the patient's head, the application of the drill. It can't take that long to make a hole in someone's head and thread in a drain for the accumulating blood, but it felt like we stood there for hours, me holding the pager and writing down numbers when it beeped, him blinking to keep his exhaustion away.

When he was finally done he put his right forearm up to his

forehead one last time. He set down the drill and without even looking at me took the pager along with the numbers I'd written down. He turned around to the phone on the wall behind the patient and started dialing.

Peter hangs up the phone now and our attention turns back to him. "I'm going to go back and talk to the family. Akash, you prepare." The surgical residents nod and start to leave in a group, including Akash. "I'll call you," I mouth to him, holding up the paper where his number is written down. Then I follow Peter and his medical student back down the hall to Sheila's room.

"How's Arthur's leg?" Peter asks. My husband badly broke his left tibia and fibula a couple winters before.

"It's good, hurts occasionally."

"Really?" he looks puzzled, but we've reached Sheila's room, so I can't ask him why Arthur's continuing leg soreness seems confusing. He gives the door a quick rap before opening it. I pretend the medical student isn't standing right behind me. If I ignore him he can't keep me out of the room with questions.

Sheila is half-sitting up in bed and two more people, a man and a woman, roughly Sheila's age, are also in the room. I'm guessing they're relatives.

"Does anyone else in your family have this clotting disorder?" Peter asks. It seems abrupt, but then I remember he's talked to them already. I was the one who missed that conversation.

"Well, we think our mom probably had it," the woman in the room says, "and our brother maybe, too." She glances at Sheila. "We don't hear a lot from him, though." She shakes her head. "But the rest of us are close."

The man, sitting in a lounge chair in the room's back corner and wearing a baseball cap, is half in shadow and has a thick black beard. Peering, I see that his wedding ring looks like it matches the one Sheila's sister is wearing. The brother-in-law. His baseball cap has a wrench printed on it and I can just make out the writing in the dark, FIELDS' PLUMBING. I remember a note about a family business. Maybe the three of them all work together.

Peter describes the operation Sheila will have in detail, how they'll remove part of her colon and most likely leave her with a colostomy. A colostomy is a diversion of the bowel to the wall of the abdomen. The end of Sheila's colon will be relocated to the skin of her belly and her large intestine will drain into a bag that attaches there. When I first learned about colostomies I found them unsettling, even repellant, but a nursing instructor reminded me, "Life is precious." All it does is change where the shit comes out; that is not worth dying for.

Peter explains that some colostomies are reversible and some aren't. Sheila's probably will be, but doing any surgery on her is risky because of the antiphospholipid antibody syndrome. In the end he would probably advise against restoring her bowel to its natural configuration: the potential risks of bleeding or clotting seem to permanently outweigh the benefits of returning to normal.

Then the conversation turns darker. Nothing changes in Peter's demeanor, but the things he says come across as almost cruel. "You're a smoker and you're overweight," he tells her. Both things will cause Sheila to heal more slowly than normal and she's going to have a big incision.

Then he drops the other shoe and it's a big one: "There's a twenty percent chance you won't survive this operation."

I look over at him. He's wearing a dark suit, holding a sheaf of papers in his hand. His expression hasn't changed. There's maybe a little more intensity around the eyes, but he's very clear and not impersonal. He could be a lawyer, an accountant, a corporate vice-president—anyone but a surgeon. Except that he is a surgeon.

I would not want to give Sheila such news, but he does it without flinching; he just says it. He is a kind man, a good doctor. I know both those things. How does it feel to tell someone there's a one in five chance the operation she is preparing for will kill her?

I could ask him, probably will ask him at some point, but I already know he won't tell me the truth. Instead he'll say he was thinking about what's for lunch, or remembering some joke one of the nurses in ICU told him earlier, or that he'd kill for a cup of bad coffee.

Myself, I feel charged up. I guess it's an adrenaline rush, the same one that started when I heard we would give Mr. Hampton Rituxan, and that ramped up even more when the radiologist called me about Sheila. What if we kill him and can't save her?

Peter finishes talking and Sheila starts to cry quietly. He's already on his way out, trailed by the medical student. We're all too damn busy. I'm sure this emergency has been shoved into a completely packed schedule. He has no time to be gentle.

Sheila looks as if she's having an internal struggle. She is afraid, but is also telling herself not to be a baby, to stop crying. I want to validate her more vulnerable feelings.

"This is big," I say, hoping that doesn't just increase her anxiety and wishing I could stay in the room with her and her family. Instead I hand her the Kleenex box and rush out after Peter. "I'll be back," I announce, "I want to ask him a few more questions out in the hall."

At the nurse's station Peter is on the phone with Dr. Martin, Sheila's physician who felt out of his element on morning rounds. "Can we give FFP? Platelets?" He wants to use a blood product that promotes clotting—fresh frozen plasma, a transfusion of platelets—to make surgery safer and faster. But when Peter gets off the phone he reports, with just a touch of irritation in his voice, that according to Martin transfusions will not speed up Sheila's clotting time; we all just have to wait.

Peter's too polite to say anything like this directly, but I suspect he feels blown off, as if the cancer doc, already bothered by having a patient with an unusual blood disorder, is even less inclined to be thoughtful now that she's been found to have a surgical problem. He could also just be frustrated there is no quicker fix than waiting.

We don't talk about Dr. Martin, but we do talk about what will most likely happen to Sheila and when. I need the process to be clear so that I can explain it to Sheila and her family.

Before I return to Sheila's room I ask the secretary to call maintenance and make sure they got the new shower curtain for Candace. I haven't seen anyone on the floor but I might have missed him.

"Shower curtain? They were brand-new a month ago. These are the new ones that, um, you know, keep off germs."

"I gotta go," I tell her, frowning just enough to look hang dog without being pathetic. "Can you just call for me?"

"If you stop making that awful face," she says.

I laugh out loud. "Deal!" Then I head back down the hall and see Sheila's intern in our secondary computer room off the hallway.

"Hey," I say, and she nods at me. "Surgery's been here. Peter Coyne, do you know him? We're increasing her fluids to 175, normal saline—"

She interrupts me. "It's not my case anymore."

"What?"

"She's switched over to surgical. She's not my patient."

"Oh." I wonder why no one told me. It's the kind of change that should go on our whiteboard, too, but often gets forgotten.

"I like hearing how she's doing, so thanks."

"Sure. No problem."

I go back into Sheila's room. She's quietly crying and her shoulders gently shake as one tear after another slides down her face. She looks at me with that same guilelessness I noticed this morning. Her sister, however, won't look at me at all.

"She thinks it's wrong for doctors to give odds like that," the husband says, indicating his wife. He's leaned forward out of the shadow so that I can see his face. Above his bushy black beard his eyes look pained. His thick fingers are spread out straight on his solid thighs and he holds his torso stiffly. "She thinks it does more harm than good."

Sheila's sister is right, of course she's right, but she's wrong, too. If the worst happens isn't it better to have some forewarning, to know before surgery that her sister may not come out of the OR alive? Wouldn't we all want to know that? Or is that just me, stubbornly wedded to the truth no matter how painful it is or how remote? The odds are in Sheila's favor, but it's not my sister who's going under the knife; maybe if it were I wouldn't want to know the risks, either.

"Yes," I say. There's no need to convince her that Peter's honesty was ethically correct or even essential for informed consent. Sheila will get the operation and she will probably survive it. Why argue about the right or wrong thing to say? Fixing Sheila's perforated bowel will threaten her life but if we do not fix it she will die.

I say nothing else and Sheila's sister turns around to look at me. Her face is drawn and she's dark where Sheila is pale, but their features are very similar: the same round eyes, the same cute button nose. Right now, more than anything, the entire family needs someone to trust.

One summer when I was a kid a group of us were playing outside—me, my brother, the Allen boys, my best friend Erica—and it started to lightly rain, but only in small, separated patches. In southern Missouri, where I grew up, summers are hot and the rain felt good, but it was unusual, startling, how it fell in one spot for just a minute, then stopped, moved a couple of yards and started up again.

We ran after the rain, chased it, wanted to always be under it as sunlight glinted through the drops, making a lattice of light out of the bursts of gently falling water. "It's over here," one of us would call out, running to the rain. "No, now it's here," someone else would say, heading off in the opposite direction: "I've got it! I've got it!"

There were no interruptions to this summer idyll, no adults asking what we were doing, just us kids, breathless, moving fast. Did it last for five minutes? Ten? It wasn't any longer than that, but I can recall the joy I felt. How rare—the chance to catch a rainstorm.

> To see a World in a Grain of Sand
> And a Heaven in a Wild Flower
> Hold Infinity in the palm of your hand
> And Eternity in an hour

William Blake wrote those lines more than a century ago and he was on to something. It's not exaggerating to say that Sheila could be dead tomorrow. Today this is the storm we chase: the infinite potential of Sheila's continuing life, held in the hand of the hospital. As a child I experienced only wonder while running after flashes of rain; I saw a world, a heaven. Now, grown-up, I try to draw on my child's sense of awe and commitment as I help Sheila confront, perhaps, the end of her time on earth.

She will have pain, her blood pressure will need watching, and her blood itself has already been revealed as untrustworthy. Getting the timing right is critical, so I'll be following the rain, but looking for the light. I believe there will be light if only I can find it in the storm.

I sit down in the chair next to Sheila's bed and take hold of her hand. It's soft and warm and she gives me a sad smile. Her sister reaches over and uses her own hand to wipe Sheila's tears. Then she, the sister, takes hold of Sheila's other hand. "Here's what will happen," I tell them. "We'll allow six hours minimum for the Argatroban to clear, then we'll draw labs to check Sheila's clotting time and see where we are. Surgery tonight, but it's impossible to say what time even approximately; there are too many unknowns." I tell them Peter is a good doctor and will do an excellent job. I tell them I'll be with Sheila, and the two of them, until she leaves the floor and afterwards she'll go to the ICU because she'll need the close attention intensive care provides.

I hold infinity in the palm of my hand, and eternity in the next few crucial hours.

CHAPTER 6

Paperwork

The time I spent with Sheila, her sister, and brother-in-law feels like one of the most important things I will do today, but it doesn't show up on any of my electronic to-do lists. We need a menu that includes the option: spent time comforting patient with life-threatening diagnosis. But nothing that empathy-intense gets included in our required paperwork.

A lot of what nurses document is strictly CYA, as in Cover Your Ass. We record most of what we do on paper, or more typically, in the computer, including proof that we're complying with all the regulatory requirements for hospitals. The morning assessment on every patient—what I heard when I listened to their lungs and heart, how their skin looked and whether they are moving their bowels—must be charted in addition to all medications given. Pain medicine, like the Dilaudid I gave Sheila, gets charted on a series of menus that specify where she feels pain, rate her pain from one to ten (based on me asking her, with ten being the 'worst pain ever'), and say whether the pain is aching, burning, cramping, stabbing, shooting, or another of the fifteen different descriptive options. Patient care—looking after Sheila, Dorothy, Richard Hampton, and Candace—is heart and soul, but these days, charting pulls nurses away from the bedside more and more.

Now's a good time to catch up on my charting, though, because lunch is being delivered. The woman taking in trays catches my eye. "Fields is NPO now. Is that right?"

"Yes. Thank you." NPO: short for *nil per os*, which is Latin for "nothing by mouth."

I try to chart my meds on the computer as I go along since that makes it less likely I'll forget something. Charting my morning assessments before the morning is actually over is a goal every shift and I did Mr. Hampton's and Dorothy's, except, I realize, shaking my head, I never even did an assessment on Candace, much less charted it. She just got here and she's energetically cleaning her room so it's likely she's fine, but I need to listen to her heart and lungs, formally ask how she's doing, and then record all that on the computer.

Before Candace, though, I need to finish my notes on Sheila, particularly since my morning assessment was wrong in crucial ways. I put in a note about her perf, including when and how I found out about it. Then I go to a different screen and I pull up the spreadsheet where we document our daily clinical observations. Bowel sounds? I didn't hear them, but didn't think that silence through. The documentation seems pointless in light of what her real problem is. Neither I nor the medical staff nor the nurses and doctors in the emergency department, paid the right kind of attention to what was happening in Sheila's bowel, but our mistaken observations have to be checked off on multiple drop-down menus so that the record is complete. I do understand why such thoroughness matters legally, but I sometimes wonder if sadists designed our software. It should not be easier to order a sweater from Lands End than to chart on my patients, but it is. Click, scroll, type, enter. Here's the menu with twenty choices, none of them the one I need. Here's the point where I need information from two different screens, but there's no way to toggle between them. Here's the screen with thirty discrete options to check, but the window it opens up only shows me five at a time. New lab results, X-rays, CT scans, MRIs: none of those generate an alert and the screen is full of minute icons, some of which represent functions I don't use or even understand.

Finally I finish up Sheila's assessment and check it off on my papers. Then I look for new orders and see that Dorothy's discharge paperwork isn't yet in the system. I look at my watch: 1:00 p.m. Not bad, except that I need to chart on Candace. It's frustrating to end a shift and then stay late doing the day's charting. "If it isn't charted it isn't done" is the mantra we hear over and over again in school.

Another one of the oncology fellows is suddenly next to my medcart, holding the written order for Mr. Hampton's Rituxan. Since the fellows are learning to be oncologists they write the chemo orders, but with more or less supervision from the attendings depending on how long they've been around. This fellow is visibly pregnant. She continues to wear heels to work, and I admire her commitment to style even though I would wear flats myself. I take the order and stare at it. "We're really doing this?"

"I know—he doesn't look so good. We are keeping it at a steady rate—not increasing the dose over time. That'll make it easier for him to tolerate."

I nod, ignoring that fluttery feeling in my stomach.

"And we got permission to give it inpatient?" Rituxan falls under one of the odder billing rules in the U.S. health care system. Reimbursement for the drug is much smaller if patients receive it in the hospital, rather than in an outpatient clinic, and it's an expensive drug. I've had patients transferred from their inpatient room to our outpatient clinic simply to receive a dose of Rituxan, but it can be given to admitted patients if the medical director of the oncology division approves that decision, and Mr. Hampton's frailty is a good argument for infusing the drug in the hospital. If he reacts badly to it we have the ability to respond more fully than a clinic could.

She gives a dry laugh that sounds like a snort. "If he's going to get this drug it has to be here. He's too sick to get it outside a hospital."

We look at each other and both raise our eyebrows, frowning. "Hey, thanks for bringing it over so quickly—I know you're in clinic and," I wave my hand toward her belly, "pregnant."

"Yeah, well, it was slow today," she says, "Can you believe it?"

"Maybe we're curing cancer!"

"Wouldn't that be great." She turns to go and then turns back to me. "I'm on call this afternoon and then it's Bruce this evening, so if anything goes wrong . . ."

"I'll call you."

She lowers her voice and leans in to me. "I'll explain to Bruce in sign-out. And just call us; don't call the house staff. The intern wouldn't know what to do."

"Got it. Fingers crossed," I say, holding up my left hand with the first two fingers twined around each other. It may be dumb, but it makes me feel better.

Mr. Hampton's weakness, his difficulty breathing, his confusion are all on my mind. Will we save him or push him closer to death? You can only know what you know, a wise friend told me, but so much is on the line here in the hospital I sometimes want to know more than I can.

I pick up the chemo form and really look at it. Chemotherapy orders continue to come on paper. The thinking is that the drugs are so strong, the regimens so specific, that a physical copy of the entire order needs to be in the patient's chart as well as entered into the computer. I like the tactility of paper, feeling it between my fingers, hearing it snap and crinkle when bent, running the tip of my finger over the slight indentations left by the fellow's careful printing.

Sheila's call light goes on. The clock's running on getting this chemo order to pharmacy, but I've got a little time since Mr. Hampton's son won't be here before three.

Sheila's room is so still it seems airless. I peer into the dimness and consciously relax my face before I speak. Sheila looks defeated, exhausted from crying. "Is your belly hurting you?"

She shakes her head. Her sister sits next to her, holding her hand. "We'd like to see a minister," she says, and her voice catches, "just in case."

"Right." This is an easy request. I call the hospital operator and ask her to page the pastor on call.

"I'll check your pressure while I'm here." I feel a flash of guilt that I hadn't checked it earlier, then suppress that feeling as I grab the cuff from its plastic holder on the wall and take the stethoscope down from the hook behind the bed. As I stick the ends of the stethoscope in my ears Sheila and her sister watch me trustingly. The trace of tears on Sheila's face makes her look like a child. "We need to know that her blood pressure is staying up. I'll be quick." I wrap the cuff around her arm, pump up the bulb, and slide the bell of the yellow disposable stethoscope under the cuff. Up the arrow goes on the dial and I see the cuff tighten around Sheila's arm. As quickly as I can I let it out and hear the first click—her systolic pressure—then the count down of five quieter clicks, the Karatkoff sounds, and the louder final click. I let the rest of the air out with a shoosh and take the stethoscope out of my ears, unwrap the Velcro cuff from her arm.

"Is it OK?" her sister asks me.

"Yes." I purse my lips. "One sixty over one hundred."

"But that's high, right?"

"Yes, but high is good right now considering the operation

she'll be having. With a perforation and major abdominal surgery coming up, a blood pressure that's abnormally low would be more troubling." I'm ready to explain more, but I see that tears hover in her eyes. She blinks them away and her features become fluid as she struggles to hold in her grief. Hearing more medical details from me right now will probably not help.

I bend down beside the bed and take hold of Sheila's sister's free hand. "I'll send in the pastor as soon as she gets here."

The brother-in-law surprises me with a question as I'm going out the door. "Do you think it was the ambulance ride that did this? All that bouncing around? She said it was rough."

I stop to consider that. "I don't think so." Lots of people ride in ambulances without having their intestines perforate. "It more likely has to do with her clotting problem and the trouble she was having with her medication." He nods, then leans back into the chair and I lose him to the corner's darkness.

I look at Sheila and her sister. "I'll be back. Call me if you need anything for pain or . . . anything else."

People react so differently to distress. Sheila and her family could be furious, focusing on our failure to do a CT scan right away, to start the anti-clotting drug without understanding why her belly hurt. They're not being like that, though; they're mostly suffering in silence. That's their portion and it makes my life easier, but I wonder if it serves them. Those who bear up, demanding little, are the reverse version of patients such as Candace Moore. Candace is a wounded Fury—hurt and wanting help but focused also on justice and some desire for revenge. It's impossible for Candace to simply endure. She lashes out at everything and everyone, unsure whom to trust since it's really her disease holding most of the cards in the hospital. I wish I had more time to sit and hold every patient's hand. To really listen. I think it would make a difference for Candace as well as Sheila. I really do.

There was an afternoon when I had time. My patient, a married man in his sixties, healthy and fit except for having leukemia, had received a cord blood transplant and it hadn't taken. That is, he'd gotten an infusion of stem cells from a stranger's— a baby's—umbilical cord, but the graft of cells failed. The day eventually arrived when we knew, without a doubt, that the treatment was unsuccessful and we also knew that his cancer would recur and he would die of it. He'd fought cancer and lost, and the inevitability of it all was making him bitter. He had a lot of living he still wanted to do.

The afternoon all this became undeniably clear to us and to him, I was his nurse and I was very lucky that it was one of those rare afternoons when I wasn't all that busy, although I can't remember why. Maybe my other patients were off the floor at tests. Maybe they were on the upside of treatment and weren't that sick. Maybe they were all taking long restorative naps.

I spent a lot of the middle part of that day in Joe's room. I didn't do much, and then again I did all I could: I listened. Sometimes people just need to talk, to say the same things over and over and over. I listened while Joe did that.

"It's not that I'm angry the treatment failed, just disappointed.

"I wish I'd had a better idea this might not work.

"It's no one's fault, but I hoped for a better result."

He would stop, then start up again where he'd left off: "What if we hadn't had that two-week delay at the start—could that have made the difference?"

I said almost nothing. He needed only a witness to his suffering. He was in the impossible position of standing on a train track waiting for the train he knew would eventually run him down, and no one he knew could be with him that day—not his wife or a neighbor or friend—but I was there silently listening as he tried, by talking, to turn his pain into a story he could accept.

At the end of the shift I told Helen, the same night-shift nurse I'd talked to this morning about Ray Mason, that I'd spent a lot of time in Joe's room listening. I felt as if I'd had it too easy, but at the same time I was exhausted. There's nothing easy about helping someone start the journey from life to death. "They also serve who only stand and wait," the poet Milton said. It's a line I often hear in my head at work, where standing and waiting can be the best service we offer.

Today is not that day, though.

My phone rings. "Theresa, just wondering when you're going to have that Rituxan order?" It's pharmacy. "We want to get it going ASAP since they're not increasing the rate. The docs would rather it didn't run all night long."

The chemo order is lying on my medcart where I left it and I and another nurse have to verify it before the paper goes to pharmacy. "Yeah. Sorry. I just got it; I'll start my check now."

"It's fine. We've got a lot of chemo to do for the other on-cology floor and wanted to make sure we finished your Rituxan first."

"Right. Thanks, Bobby." So many needs; I'd better get this done.

Focus: the fellow's calculation of the BSA or body surface area is the first thing to check. We calculate from a verified height and weight, which requires two nurses to weigh and measure Mr. Hampton together. That must have been done yesterday. I double-check by looking it up on the computer—it's there—and then double-check the math, multiplying Mr. Hampton's height in centimeters by his weight in kilograms, dividing by 3,600, and taking the square root of that number. The answer comes out in meters squared, which makes no sense and yet it's what we do.

All of this is just arithmetic, but mistakes slip in. Fellows round down instead of up, use an old weight, plug the numbers into the non-customary formula—these kinds of errors and others have been detected by nurses reviewing chemotherapy orders. The drugs are biohazards, so the dose has to be pre-cise: more than enough to cure the patient's disease might be too much for the patient's body to tolerate since many of these drugs are toxic enough at the predetermined safe doses.

I use the calculator on my computer desktop and this time the numbers for the BSA and the ordered dose of Rituxan are correct. Good. Now I need to make sure the ordered dose and timing of Mr. Hampton's Rituxan match the treatment plan specific to his disease. Pulling up chemoregimens.com on my computer (luckily the website is not blocked today) I go to lymphoma and easily find Mr. Hampton's regimen. Harder are the moments when I can't find the correct doses listed and a call to the fellow yields the information that they're using a novel protocol taken from brand-new research. "The article's in the front of the chart," the fellow will say, helpfully, but why didn't she or he just tell me at the start? Often the docs are too busy to think of that detail, but it may also be because MDs have little idea what nurses actually do when we check chemo orders. Do they know that we perform our own independent verification of the math and the ordered regimen? Nurses and doctors—our work is often invisible to each other.

I'm at the final step: I need another nurse to redo my verification. I walk up the hall and there's Beth at the nurses' station. I feel uncertain about asking her to help me since I know her daughter's trip to Kandahar is on her mind, but she sees the order sheet in my hand and says, "You need a checker?"

"Do you have time?"

"Being busy is good," she says. And then she laughs, "But then you may have to double-check my math. I'm a little preoccupied." She's joking; I know how careful she is.

"Any word?" I ask quietly.

"No," she says, not looking up. She's pulled a small calculator out of her pocket and is already punching in numbers. "And I've decided it's just too early to worry!" she says, briefly glancing up, but she presses her lips together in a hard line as she compares the calculations.

I see Ray Mason sitting up on a stretcher on the opposite

side of the nurses' station, near the main door to the floor. He must be on his way to a test. I realize it's past noon and even though I talked to his wife, Liz, in the hall I haven't yet gone by to say hi to him. Leaving Beth to her work I walk over.

"Hey," he says. He's taken out his nose and ear piercings and looks vulnerable without them. I bend down to the stretcher to hug him.

Something in my face must give away my concern for him, because he says, "It's cool. What will be will be." He says it in a rush, with little feeling, almost like a mantra. Well, why not invoke karma? There's nothing else he can do.

"What happened?"

"Just started feeling more and more tired. Got a blood test. Have to do a marrow, but . . ." he shrugs. The relapse isn't 100 percent confirmed until leukemia cells are detected in a sample of his bone marrow, but he's resigned to it.

"The thing is, my brother, the super-conservative, will be my donor. I'm worried I'll end up being like him." I look at Ray; I can't tell if he's kidding or not and decide to go with "not kidding."

"No!" I tell him, "That's ridiculous!"

"I don't know," he says, "I'll be getting his entire immune system."

"Nah," I tell him. "Your personality won't change—just your blood cells."

The escort who's taking Ray to whatever test he's having steps up to the stretcher. He's ready to roll.

"Hey," I say, "I'm sorry." They take off toward the elevator and Ray, with his back to me on the stretcher, raises one hand in the air and waves it at me without turning around, friendly, but dismissive. He doesn't want my pity.

I met Ray for the first time during the follow-up chemotherapy to his initial treatment—what we call consolidation. He'd brought a guitar to the hospital and the live music on the floor seemed to free time from its usually strict moorings. Ray's signature line was "It's cool" and one evening I volunteered to hang his dose of chemo because Nora, his nurse, was busy with another patient's emergency.

My taking Nora's place didn't faze Ray at all. He sat on the bed, bald, calm, looking like a young Buddha. He seemed to have a deep belief in fate, the idea that life works out the way it should. It makes sense that if you crossed the heedlessness of a firefighter with the anarchism of a punk rocker the result would be a person acutely aware of life's randomness.

I can't remember what Ray and I talked about, but I remember the feeling that I could breathe in his room, really breathe, as if I'd already pushed his particular rock to the top of the hill and had nothing more to do than look around.

The next summer, after Ray finished consolidation, he went back to work as a firefighter. I know this because he came to visit one day on the floor. We knew him as a patient, bald, stuck in the hospital, weak, coping. The day he stopped by it felt as though Odysseus from Homer's *Odyssey*, that most well-known of lost travellers, was visiting the underworld of his own volition. Well-muscled, trim, with a full head of thick brown hair and a lingering smell of summertime sweat, he explained that he'd spent the afternoon at the firefighter training grounds crawling around in tunnels.

He knew, he said, that some of the guys he worked with thought he wouldn't be able to come back to the job, that he would have to prove he could do it. So he did: lifting weights, navigating dark tunnels with only a flashlight and his wits, carrying the heavy equipment he would need to save lives.

Odysseus visited Hades seeking knowledge of the future from the prophet Tiresias. Ray came to us as a bearer of the rarest and most precious knowledge to be had on an oncology floor: that people make it. The miracle of oncology is that patients confront their own possible death, and move on.

To keep Ray and Candace moving, they both will receive stem cell transplants. Candace will have her own cells infused. Ray will take donated cells from his brother the Republican. Different diseases require different treatments. Ray has the harder road, since receiving another person's stem cells can cause a lot more problems afterwards than getting one's own back. For both of them, transplant day will arrive with a sense of anticipation and a bit of low-key fanfare.

Candace's cells, harvested earlier and then frozen solid, will be thawed in a water bath by the cell technician who attends every transplant. The numbers on each bag will be checked and double-checked to make sure she receives only her own cells. As each bag is thawed the nurse will hook it up to Candace's central line and let it flow in just like any other blood product. The preservative used on the cells, called DMSO, could be dangerous, though. A few unlucky patients have a potentially fatal allergic reaction to it and we have no way of knowing in advance who those patients may be. Because of the risk posed by DMSO we put all patients receiving an autologous stem cell transplant on a heart monitor, make sure to have oxygen tubing and suction equipment in the room, take vital signs every five minutes, and stay with them at all times. I even give my phone up to the charge nurse.

This is nurses' work and it's a privilege to do it. It's not every day you get to give someone her life back by hanging an IV, checking some vitals, and making sure she continues to breathe deeply since the body eliminates DMSO through respiration.

The DMSO also produces a distinct odor. Some people smell garlic, others tomato soup. For me it's creamed corn. It's not a nice scent, but it is a joyful one. Yeast proofing in water smells like nothing anyone would want to eat, but, with proper mixing and baking, turns flour, sugar, and water into bread. Similarly, an aroma of DMSO, even days after an auto, will make me recoil and, on reflection, smile because it tells me another patient is on the road to survival.

When Ray gets his transplant he won't have any worries about DMSO, because the cells from his brother will be fresh. He'll be carefully monitored, but the transplant itself is relatively risk-free; the trouble for him, if it comes, will begin later when his body may attack the "graft," or infusion of his brother's cells. The really nice thing will be if his brother can be in the room during the transplant. I had this happen once. The patient's brother finished donating cells in the morning and the transplant took place in the afternoon, so he got to see his cells infused; got to see a new shot at life, donated by him, flow into his own brother's veins. It's trendy in some restaurants now to serve beef marrow and people say it's delicious. I wouldn't know. Having given the stem cell portion of this precious substance to patients as a lifesaver I can't imagine eating it, but I can attest to its beauty: deep red, iridescent with flashes of white and pinks.

We say "Happy Birthday" to all transplant patients. The stem cells they receive—whether their own or someone else's— are needed because we use very high doses of chemotherapy to wipe out their own marrow's ability to produce stem cells. The transplant is technically a rescue therapy after they've gotten enough chemo to kill their disease, but I like the rebirth analogy better. If donated cells differ in blood type from the patient's own, that person's blood type will actually change after transplant and engraftment. I used to think blood type was as fixed as eye color or having dimples, but it isn't. It can change, does change, as a side-effect of the treatment given to save someone's life.

Beth gives me back the Rituxan order. "That's my call light," she says, hearing the insistent beep and checking the screen at the nurses' station for a room number. "Mr. Parrish probably needs help to the bathroom."

I check that we both signed the form in the right place, dated it, wrote down the time: 13:45. I like that we use military time in the hospital; it avoids confusion. I glance over the order sheet one more time, then leave it in the bin for pharmacy.

There's a pre-operation assessment that I need to fill out for Sheila and I'll do that back at my medcart.

Before I start the pre-op form, I check on her. I open the door slowly and peer into the dark. "Pain?" I ask her. She nods, just barely.

"I'll get you some more Dilaudid."

Inside the locked room where we keep our narcotics I punch my code into the Pyxis machine, just as I did this morning, look up Sheila's name and get the dose of Dilaudid I need. Back at my medcart I draw it up and dilute it as usual.

I chart the med, guessing at the number on the one-to-ten pain scale since it's subjective and I know she needs it. The few times I've been asked to rate my own pain from one to ten I've found it inaccurate and unhelpful. Hurts some, hurts a lot, and oh-my-God give me relief now seems like a more appropriately human scale.

In the room I hold up the syringe, saying nothing. I prepare the IV port and slowly push the drug in while I explain how to best manage pain. "If you can, call me in before it gets so bad; we call that 'staying ahead of the pain.' Pain is not physiologically neutral. It stresses the immune system, interrupts sleep, can delay healing. I can also get your dose increased if you need more relief."

Sheila grimaces, then nods while closing her eyes, taking a sharp breath in. I unscrew the used syringe and attach another filled syringe. "This is saline," I say. "If I push this in in fast it will make sure the drug gets into your system as quickly as possible." I probably don't need to do that since she's got IV fluids running in at such a fast rate, but why not? It makes me feel like I'm doing everything possible for her. I look at the one-quarter full bag of saline that's running now; she'll need a new one soon. That's a small something I can do as well.

"I paged a minister," I say. "It seems like it's taking her a while to get here so I'll page again. Sometimes it's good to be the squeaky wheel."

The sister actually smiles, but Sheila catches a sound in her throat. The brother-in-law is sitting closer to the two of them than he had been, but he has his head down and is staring intently into his lap. He's unreadable.

When I leave a patient's room I try to always ask, "Is there anything I can get for any of you?" We have soda, ice water, crackers, bread for toast, peanut butter. This time, though, I don't ask. I throw the empty syringes away, pull off my latex gloves, and drop them in the trash.

The door quietly latches shut behind me and I want to leave, to walk off the floor. I want five minutes to collect my thoughts, go get some tea, maybe, not feel responsible, when—

"There you are!"

It's Candace. She's put a hospital gown over her sleek black yoga pants and has another gown on backward, ensuring that her back is completely covered.

"Aren't you supposed to listen to my lungs and ask me how I'm doing? Isn't that part of being in the hospital?"

I swallow. Transitioning from Sheila to Candace feels like turning inside out: *Umgekehrt*, a German word for "upside down," "confused." It fits. "Right." I offer a weak smile, like a cup of half-brewed tea, the one I don't have time for. "I wanted to let you get settled in first."

"Or maybe you just forgot," she says. Her words are accusing, but her tone is neutral and her face looks pleasant enough.

"Well, how about now?" I hold out my hands, palms up, like a used car salesman ready to make a deal.

"My cousin just left, so now's good. She's coming back but I needed a few things. And we used up almost all of the Clorox wipes."

I follow her back into the room and pull the disposable stethoscope down from her IV pole. The overlapping gowns billow around her like a cape. Only Candace could make a hospital gown look that stylish.

She sits lightly on the edge of the bed, collects her long hair and, looking down, pulls it around behind her neck and over her right shoulder so that a tuft of thick black hair rests on her right chest. Suddenly I see the person she probably is outside the hospital—energetic, aggressive, but personable. Here, inside, all that gets channeled into an unstinting wariness.

"You look so good," I tell her. And it's true. She's slim with small muscles that are well toned. Her long hair is her hair. It may yet fall out from chemo, but it's now jet black, thick and shiny in the light.

"Deep breaths," I say, as I move the stethoscope around on her back, then to her upper chest and sides. Her breathing is soft, easy.

"Your lungs are clear," I tell her, placing the stethoscope on her heart and reaching down with my right hand to check the pulse on her left wrist. The blood flow is steady and strong. I squat down and check her ankles for swelling, ask her to lie back and listen to her belly. Unlike Sheila's, Candace's bowel is loud and healthy and the sound of gurgling reassures me.

Abraham Verghese, the physician and writer, speaks eloquently about the value of touch in health care. During a lecture here in Pittsburgh he explained that when doctors examine patients by physically touching them the patients feel more thoroughly cared for than if they had only been asked questions and observed. That reaction makes sense since when we're ill it's usually our bodies that are sick and hold the details of our affliction; a doctor intuitive enough to diagnose from touch is not just appealing, but reassuring.

Nurses touch patients all the time, typically not to make diagnoses, since that's not what we officially do, but to gather information and to help—with going to the bathroom, bathing, walking, eating, managing pain, figuring out if someone's taking a turn for the worse. Touch connects the essential humanness of nurse and patient, reminding me that we are two people with a shared mission: healing, if we can. The image of a mother placing the back of her hand on a child's feverish forehead is indelible because it communicates, "I can feel how you feel when you are ill."

I take the ends of the stethoscope out of my ears. "You're healthy," I tell Candace.

"Except for my cancer!"

"Right. Except for your cancer. It's not fair, is it?"

I point to her right side just below the tail of black hair covering her clavicle. Three plastic tubes dangle from a holder inserted in her chest. "That's the line that isn't working?"

"Um-huh."

"Let me call IR, see if I can get a time for when they'll be ready for you."

"Oh thanks." Turning away, she swings her legs around and gets up on the other side of the bed, starts rummaging in one of her suitcases, but her "thanks" seemed sincere.

"You're—" The door bursts open and the fellow, Yong Sun, walks into the room looking slightly lost. I was just about to say, "You're welcome," when his entrance interrupted me.

Whirling around, Candace looks him up and down through narrowed eyes, "Who are you?" she demands. She's got a point. People in white coats go in and out of hospital rooms all the time, often without knocking or even saying their names. No one would like that and, unlike a lot of patients, Candace doesn't hide her discomfiture.

I should stay and help out the fellow but I don't have time. There are too many other priorities: call IR, start the pre-op checklist, confirm the timing of the Rituxan with pharmacy, repage the pastor, look in on Mr. Hampton and see whether he has finally woken up.

I do this all day long: run through a mental checklist that changes unpredictably. Of course I have things written down, but nurses spend the shift recalibrating the tasks we have and their urgency. Doing an assessment on Candace right when she gets here? Not that pressing. Monitoring Sheila's blood pressure more than ordered—very important.

An old animated sketch on *Sesame Street* shows a little girl being instructed by her mother to bring home some basic groceries: a loaf of bread, a container of milk, and a stick of butter. The mother offers to write down the list, but the little girl is sure she can remember. She walks to the store repeating, "A loaf of bread, a container of milk, and a stick of butter," over and over, and she does remember once she's there, but only by bringing her mother's exact words to mind. In the hospital I'm like that little girl on my way to the store, except the trip lasts twelve hours and the items I have to remember are much more varied and potentially consequential.

The computer tells me that Dorothy's discharge paperwork is ready to complete; she can leave after I've done my part. I push Candace and the well-intentioned but awkward and difficult-to-understand fellow to the back of my mind along with all my other to-dos and head up to the nurses' station. Let me see how quickly I can get Dorothy out of here. Leaving the hospital to go home always makes people glad.

CHAPTER 7

No Time for Lunch

Suddenly I'm dizzy. I look at my watch: 1:45 p.m. I usually don't feel this way until after 2:00, but I haven't had a morning snack except for those few saltines and Dorothy's candy. The dizziness will pass, but then simple things will start to make less sense. I'm not unsafe when I'm hungry, just slow, and I'll get slower the longer I wait to eat.

I'll have lunch. Dorothy's discharge can wait a few more minutes and the pastor usually lets us know when she gets here so I won't miss her if I'm off the floor.

Lunch is touchy for a lot of nurses. We don't get paid for the thirty minutes when we supposedly eat, but there's rarely staff to cover our patients, so most of us work through lunch without being paid for that time. Class-action lawsuits have been filed on behalf of nurses not getting paid for a lunch break we never take, but the practice, at least from what I hear, is common.

Even when there's an official way for nurses to note that we didn't get a lunch break and should be paid for the time, the hospital may subtly dissuade nurses from putting in a claim for every non-lunch. I worked a year at my first job before I even learned I should be paid for that time. Labor laws say that lunch is thirty minutes of uninterrupted time, but on my floor that's an uncommon abundance of time to eat, so legally pretty much every nurse I work with should be paid for lunch for every shift. Three million nurses in America. How much money do hospitals save by not paying nurses for the thirty-minute lunch break we more often than not work through?

Not to mention the physical toll of hunger. Glucose is the only form of food energy our brains can use, so if I don't eat my brain is deprived of fuel. I spend the shift going from room to room, lifting patients, pushing carriers, moving beds, raising IV poles up and down. All that uses energy. If I don't eat, the tank gets low—simple physiology.

To be clear: I'm not a martyr. I would love to pass my patients off to a lunch-nurse for a full thirty minutes and really get a break. But no lunch nurse exists on my floor and I don't like taking on another nurse's four patients while managing my own, then asking that same nurse to take on my four patients so that I can eat. Another four patients, even for half an hour, could be overwhelming or, worst of all, unsafe.

Now, though, my patients are stable and I need to eat. No one else is in the break room, so I turn off the wide-screen TV. After all the pings and beeps and buzzes and alarms on the floor I want silence.

Grabbing my lunch out of the refrigerator, I sit down and feel the physical effort of the day. I'd like to make a cradle of my arms, lay my head down on the table, close my eyes. But food comes first. I eat my turkey sandwich quickly, reminding myself to chew and take deep breaths between bites. I wash it down with ice water, sipped through a straw.

Swallow. Drink. Breathe. Bite. Chew. Breathe. Swallow.

I start to feel it: my blood sugar rising. My head clears and I blink a few times. There's nothing like food when you're hungry.

There's a knock on the door and Maya, an aide, pokes her head in.

"Hey, I know you're eating."

"No. It's OK," I gesture at the empty plastic bag and crumbs on the table. "I'm done."

"Well, it's Candace Moore."

"Uh-hunh?"

She starts counting on her fingers, holding up her index finger first: "She wants to know where she can get extra hangers and," now her middle finger, "if the water pressure in the shower can be increased."

"The water pressure?"

The aide nods. She raises her ring finger. "And she says to thank you for the new shower curtain."

"Oh, they replaced it." I smile, even though it's only a shower curtain. "Soooo, did she take a shower?"

Maya shrugs in a casual I've-got-no-idea way. "Her cousin said the water pressure wasn't good." She moves into the break room and lets the door close behind her, rests her back on it. "I said I would come tell you because I wanted to get out of the room. She is intense!"

We burst out laughing. This is absurd and yet also not. "Well, Candace is keeping us honest. By the time she leaves, the hospital will be perfect."

"Right." The aide is not convinced. "But what do I tell her now?"

I don't want to leave the break room. "Tell the secretary that Candace needs more hangers." She nods. "Ask her also to call maintenance and pass on the message about the water pressure."

"Will do." She heads back out the door when her phone rings. "You're kidding. He pooped again?!" I hear her say before the door closes.

I stay sitting for a few minutes more. It would be so nice to float. But I don't float; I take the lid off my yogurt and stir it up with a spoon.

I start to think about armchairs. A grateful patient donated money to the floor to buy some comfortable armchairs for the patient rooms. It was a very nice gesture, except there was only enough money to buy six. Enough of our patients are long-term that they now know there are a few A+ armchairs in a few of the rooms, and the chairs in the rest are B- at best. The A+ armchairs are big enough, comfortable enough, and recline enough that family members who stay over can sleep in them. They say the smooth imitation leather covering feels good on your skin, or at least much better than the thick vinyl of the B- armchairs, which barely recline at all.

I'm sure that Candace would like an A+ armchair. Can I

get her one proactively? Sick people, stuck in the hospital, already operating in an environment of scarcity since they're worried their time on earth is dwindling, are especially sensitive to deprivation and comfort. Candace would be happier with a good chair in her room.

Does Dorothy have one? I mentally run my mind around Dorothy's decorated room and realize there isn't space for one. Sheila has one of the superior armchairs, though; her brother-in-law's been sitting in it all day. After Sheila goes to the OR I can offer Candace the good armchair with its built-in pillow and puffy armrests that feel like they're giving you a hug. That will work because Sheila won't come back to the floor after her operation—they'll put her in the Surgical ICU.

I take a spoonful of yogurt with my plastic hospital spoon and slide it into my mouth. This will work. *Ping-ping-ping.*

Lucy the nurse practitioner is on the phone. Very nicely, she tells me that Dorothy's husband has arrived and wants to leave as soon as possible since it's a long ride and he hates driving at night. She knows the discharge form is in the computer. Could I just finish up the paperwork and get Dorothy out of here? I sigh. But of course.

"Yup," I tell her.

"Are you eating?"

"It's OK. I'm just finishing my yogurt."

"Theresa, it can wait five minutes. Finish eating, then do the discharge."

"You're sure?"

"It's five minutes."

"Hey thanks. I'll be out in five minutes." I look at my watch. It's 1:58 p.m.

I slowly swirl my spoon around the sides of the yogurt container. "Chocolate Underground," it's called and the bittersweet of the chocolate sets off the tang of the yogurt. I turn the spoon over in my mouth to lick off the back of it and taste a burst of liquid chocolate.

"You gonna marry that spoon?" It's my friend Gloria, with spiky hair and sass she brings from her native Tennessee.

I laugh. "I'm just enjoying my yogurt before my next five and a half hours."

"Uh-huh. That's not what I saw." Now she laughs, too, goes to her locker, and starts spinning the lock.

"Hey, where are you? I haven't seen you at all today."

"Got pulled across the hall," she tilts her head. "Just came to get money so I can eat," she takes her billfold out of her locker and holds it up. "They had two call-offs so it's busy, but I only have four patients; they didn't saddle me with the extras." Gloria was sent to another oncology floor for her shift. When one unit doesn't have enough staff they sometimes request a nurse from a sister-unit that may have a nurse to spare: the oncology floors draw from one another, the ICUs share staff, etc. No nurse really likes working on a different floor, hence the negative connotations of "being pulled." Even worse, sometimes the regular staff dump an extra patient, or the more difficult patients, onto the nurse who's come to help, but our sister oncology floor didn't do that to Gloria today.

"It's good they kept you at four patients. But two call-offs?" A call-off is what we say when a nurse doesn't show up for a scheduled shift. "Call" because we use the phone to notify the floor that we won't be there. No matter the reason—death in the family or an emergency appendectomy—there are nurses who always resent call-offs, because a nurse not showing up means more work for everyone else who's there. It's telling that we don't call them sick days, only call-offs.

"Someone's car wouldn't start, and Tony's wife went into labor."

"Nice! But who's Tony? I don't know him."

"I don't think he's been there that long. We renewed CPR together—that's where I met him."

"It's a nice reason for a call-off."

"Yeah. And the charge nurse is taking patients to pick up the slack."

"Really? How's that going?"

She shuts her locker with a metallic scrape, clicks the lock closed. "She's storming around in a terrible mood, complaining about her chart audits." She laughs.

"Patients before paperwork," I say, mock-piously holding up my index finger for emphasis.

A mischievous look returns to her face. "Hey—I'll let you get back to your spoon."

I smile. "Me and the spoon are done. I've got to discharge Dorothy." I toss the plastic spoon and the yogurt container in the trash.

"She's finally going home? That's great! You back tomorrow?" I have to think about it. "Yes. You?"

"Where else would I be? Picked up an extra shift, so I'm working four twelves this week. And for that they pull me."

"Ugh. Four twelves—you're a better person than I am."

She shakes her head. "See you tomorrow. Coffee at ten? You know, if it's not crazy?" she laughs.

"Yes! I didn't have time today." She raises an eyebrow, but I don't feel like explaining. "I'll tell you tomorrow. Short version: Rituxan, a perf, and Candace Moore."

"Now, an assignment like that is just not right."

"I think everyone's a little crazy." I drop the timbre of my voice. "Did you hear about Mr. King?"

She nods somberly and I'm surprised to feel tears at the edges of my eyes. I blink them back. "Maybe being pulled is better than being here today."

"Could be," she sighs as we both move out the door. She goes to the right to take the elevator to the cafeteria while I turn to the left to get back to the floor, stopping when I remember my apple. Didn't I bring in an apple today? I'll leave it for now; maybe I can eat it later.

At the nurses' station Lucy waits for me. She puts her hand on my shoulder and gives me a small hug. Some of the nurses don't like it when she's physical, but I find it soothing—the power of touch. "Sorry I interrupted your lunch." Her manner is always distracted, as if she's half-thinking of something else, but she explains herself clearly.

"No. It's fine," I say. "She's been here for six weeks, of course they want to get home."

I sit down in front of a computer and pull up Dorothy's chart. Double-checking the list of medications Dorothy will take at home, I smile to myself when I see Omeprazole: the generic for Prilosec. Once Dorothy's home she can take her Prilosec whenever she wants.

I need a checker for the discharge instructions, so I print them out and flag down Susie, the new nurse, as she walks by. "Have time to check discharge instructions?"

She breathes out and in heavily. "Not really." In addition to the friendly couple I met this morning she's also got one of the completes, the patients who need us to bathe, dress, and feed them, and keep them clean when they go to the bathroom. That patient's wife, living in her own personal hell of guilt, anxiety, and fear, finds fault with almost everything we do. "Today, his lunch was cold and she's annoyed because the Internet connection isn't working so she can't email the family. I get it; she's the one keeping everything together, but I've called the computer HELP desk twice now and they can't fix the problem." She holds up a covered plate of food, "And I'm just now going to warm up his lunch!"

"Hey, have you eaten?"

"There's no time, Theresa."

"Go eat. You'll feel better."

She looks down at the place. "I'll just do this—"

"No. I'll do it. Give me the plate and go eat now."

"I can't."

"You can. Go. It'll be all right. I know how to use the microwave."

She nods slowly, looks at her watch again. "Fuck it." she says, handing me the plate and heading back to our break room.

Beth sidles up to me. "It's hard for the new ones. The floor's tough right now."

"I guess you're right." I watch Susie as she walks away, her curls bobbing as she moves. Does it have to be quite this hard? One in five nurses quits a first job within a year. Susie's a good nurse. I don't want her to be part of the 20 percent who leave.

Beth looks at the discharge instructions in my hand. "It looks like you need another checker, so I'm here."

I smile at her, surprised. "Thank you. I—"

"Hand 'em over," she says, reaching out. "It's Dorothy's time to go home."

"I've got to heat this up and drop it off, first—" I say, but Amy, her long blond hair down for the day, interrupts me.

"I'll do it. I like them."

"Where did you come from? I haven't seen you all day."

"I was in the conference room. I heard everything. I'm in front today, but I know that family pretty well. I'll take care of his lunch."

"It's all yours!" I tell her, handing over the plate. "I thank you and so does Susie." She shrugs and heads into our kitchen.

Turning to Beth I read from the list of drugs entered by the nurse practitioner and Beth checks it against the official list in the chart. The oncology attending will have looked over the medication record, but it's the NPs and PAs who, like the residents, do the actual work of carefully putting these lists together with correct doses and times. For Dorothy there are fifteen medications and we verify the drug, the dose, the number of doses per day, and any special instructions such as "Synthroid: Take on an empty stomach." Sometimes the prescribing practitioner who's typing up the list checks a box in error, writes down the wrong dose, or forgets to write down a dose at all. Then we page that person to get the right information, but it can take a while to pin down the correct answer. Unfortunately, the waiting patient gets angrier every minute with the—in her view—obstacle-creating nurse.

Dorothy's nurse practitioner is careful and there are no discrepancies between the different lists of prescribed meds. Beth and I take turns signing both copies of the discharge instructions and then I take one of the special discharge envelopes out of the drawer at the secretary's station and slide in Dorothy's paperwork. Dorothy will sign a separate copy and that one goes in her chart. It takes many pieces of paper to send one person home and even then the array of pills, with different doses and times, can be overwhelming. Lab tests, office visits, and scans may need to be scheduled, along with transportation to and from our outpatient cancer center. Cancer patients tend to be savvier than most. Because they often get treatment for so long, they have a lot of time to learn about their disease and how the system works, but even they sometimes feel that what they're

tasked with is unmanageable. For patients who are rarely hospitalized, who have little understanding of how the human body
works, who lack money, or simply don't read or speak English
very well, our high expectations of them as outpatients may
make any outcome but failure unlikely. All of us who work in
health care put our shoulder to that huge rock every day trying
to get the system to work. But sometimes shift after shift it feels
like the same damn rock.

I'm closing Dorothy's envelope when Nancy, the charge
nurse, lays her hand on my shoulder. "I hate to do this," she
says, "But you'll be getting another admission."

"I just got Candace Moore. And I have Rituxan and a perf."

"I know, but when Dorothy leaves you'll be down to three
and everyone else has four and I have to leave early," she says,
looking at her clipboard.

She has to leave early. *Has to?* This nurse often leaves early
while the rest of us scramble. Or maybe I just notice it, and
mind, on the days I'm especially busy. The position she has is
half regular nursing, half management and she's salaried, not
paid by the hour, so no overtime when she exceeds forty hours
per week. If the idea behind getting a salary is to elevate the staff
to a new level of professionalism it hasn't worked for this particular RN.

Truth is, she's older, has some longstanding problem with
her back, and never calls-off no matter how much her back hurts.
Her straight brown hair is cut in a severe line at shoulder-level
and her half-glasses hover halfway down her nose. She's put in
her time pushing the rock and now she's tired. I understand. Of

course I understand because I'm also tired and I've been a nurse a lot fewer years than she has.

"You know him," she says, "It's Irving Mooney." She tries to make it better: "Besides, he shouldn't be here for a while. He has to wait for an ambulance at his group home and then he's over an hour away. And they said the ambulances were all backed up."

I take the piece of paper she holds out. Worried about dropping an important ball, or worse, making a serious mistake, but also not wanting to appear a whiner I don't handle these situations well. I withdraw; suck it up.

Pride's at work here. I'm too proud to tell her the assignment feels potentially overwhelming, that I'm afraid I can't do it. I will not make myself vulnerable in front of someone who has power over me because I want to show I can do it all, that I'm that good: Theresa Brown, super nurse. If I spoke up it might make a difference—it might—but now I'll never know.

I look down at the printout. It just says 'infection' under reason for admission. "What's wrong with him?"

"I don't know." She looks down at her clipboard again. "Just call the group home," she says, "the number's right there." She points with her index finger, then walks away, making ticks with her pencil on the new paperwork she's moved on to.

I walk back to my medcart. I want to slam the admission paper down on top of it, but don't. One of the key factors in burnout, though, is employees feeling like they have little control over their work environment. That's pretty much status quo in hospitals for nurses and doctors.

Dorothy's call light comes on, its chime sounding like a reproach. "Dammit." I left her discharge papers—special envelope and all—back at the nurses' station. I should stick my head in and tell her everything's ready. But all I want is to sit down, tell the charge nurse to stay until she's scheduled just for today, and then have five minutes to eat the shiny red apple I left in the fridge.

The call light goes out and I sigh. Relief. And then my phone rings. It's Maya, the aide. "Theresa, Dorothy wants to know where her discharge papers are."

"I've got them. I'll tell her." My voice goes low.

"Are you OK?"

"I just got another admission."

And suddenly she's there, standing next to me. "Who is it?"

"Irving Mooney."

"Irving." She thinks. "He's always late; comes by ambulance."

"Yes?"

"Yes."

"Really late?"

"Hours and hours."

I smile at her. "You're lying."

"Yeah, but you're not frowning anymore." She smiles back at me.

"Hey, can you tell Dorothy I've got her paperwork ready, that I just have to get it from the nurses' station. Do you have time?"

She hesitates, then nods yes.

"Thank you!" I sing it out, smile big. A small dose of help can give me the same jolt as an afternoon coffee.

Back at the nurses' station Dorothy's papers are right where I left them. "I knew you'd be back for those, T." The secretary says. Then she lowers her voice and bends her head toward me as if she's sharing a secret. "Did Candace Moore really complain about the water pressure in her shower?"

"So I hear."

"Oh, T." she laughs. "Now that is just too much. She needs to get a little perspective."

"True that." I say. Our secretary's husband has been ill for several years with a degenerative muscular disorder. When she misses work it's usually because he's in the hospital again. She can be scatterbrained but is almost always good humored, and today I really appreciate that.

I turn and see Ray on a stretcher coming back from his test. I remember all that's at stake here: Mr. Hampton and his sometimes killer drug, Sheila and her possibly killer perf, Candace trying to save herself from what is always a killer disease. Dorothy's husband wanting to get his wife safely back home.

Nurses sometimes joke at change of shift that it was a good day if "everyone was still breathing when I left." That may sound like we set the bar way too low, but illnesses can be unconquerable. I tuck Dorothy's paperwork under my arm. It's time for her to leave this clean, well-lighted place. The armchairs in her house, I'm guessing, are not vinyl but nubby cotton and lovingly worn. There are probably shelves filled with picture frames. The candy dish ... she always kept out and full in her hospital room ... can be put away until next time, if there is a next time. I'm hoping Dorothy never graces our floor again. In all the hurly-burly, I'd forgotten, but now I remember: The most important thing of all is that everyone's alive at the end of the day.

CHAPTER 8

Duo Damsel

I dial the number of Irving's group home and a woman answers with a pleasant murmur. "Shady Oasis Center." Her words come out slowly and easily and the time she takes reminds me of how relatively unhurried people's lives seemed in southern Missouri where I grew up. "Let's see . . . Irving Mooney is going to the hospital for . . . Well, it says here—oh my goodness—it says he has an abscess . . . Oh, that must hurt." She clucks her tongue. "Poor man. He's such a nice man, too." There's silence and I realize I'm nodding my head sympathetically as she talks.

"We'll take care of him," I tell her. "Do you have any idea when he might be leaving?"

"Now, honey, I don't. All we know is they said it would be a while for the ambulance, and Irving's so patient. He doesn't mind."

"Can you call me when he leaves so I have some idea when he'll arrive?"

"I sure can. Let me just get your number . . ." She promises to call and I hang up, hoping she remembers.

Irving is a soft-voiced African American schizophrenic in his late fifties. He lives in a facility he describes as the most agreeable place he could have imagined as a home for himself. The large front porch has rocking chairs he sits in while watching the world go by, or so he's told me. I'm never sure which of Irving's memories are real since he once reported a conversation he had with an IV pump. According to him, the machine started it: "I know I'm not supposed to talk to IVs, but the pump talked to me first." So the rocking chair may not actually exist, but the idea of sitting in it makes him feel good.

You'd think schizophrenia and homelessness would be enough of a load that some sort of cosmic force of justice would keep leukemia from being added onto it, but one thing I've learned in the hospital is that life is not fair. Ill health, and especially cancer, takes all comers.

Irving's done very well with his treatment so far. We've been able to put his cancer into remission and keep it there with consolidation. Immune suppression from the chemo probably explains the abscess. A small scratch got irritated, then infected, and now needs to be treated. But there won't be a room for Irving until Dorothy is gone and housekeeping has thoroughly cleaned, so I need to get her out of here.

Sometimes that feeling of a revolving door at the hospital is exhausting. Patient flow equals income in hospitals, what I've heard administrators call "heads in beds." I wish we could occasionally slow down, but the pace won't change unless caring becomes as lucrative for hospitals as tests and procedures.

Now my phone rings and Dorothy's call light comes on at the same time. I grit my teeth and swear that giving Dorothy her paperwork will be the next thing I do even if I have to sit on the phone to quiet it, but first I do have to answer it: "Medical Oncology, this is Theresa."

It's pharmacy wanting to know if I can start the Rituxan soon because it has to go in slowly. They prepare the drug for us, so the timing of a medication depends on when they are able to mix it. "Right. I'm just waiting for the patient's son to arrive and that should be . . ." I hold the phone between my ear and shoulder and glance at my watch, "any minute now." It's almost three o'clock.

Nora, who'd teased me earlier about Candace Moore, walks by and points silently at Dorothy's call light. She holds up a bag of blood for me to see and shrugs her shoulders in a sorry-I-can't-help-you way as she moves down the hall. I hold up the special discharge envelope, showing her that I'm on top of it, and walk over to Dorothy's room, continuing to listen to Bobby in pharmacy.

I open the door to Dorothy's room with my right elbow and stand in the open doorway, finishing up my call, showing Dorothy and her husband that I have papers in my hand. "Right. Yes. I'll call you when he gets here," I confirm, punching off the phone and shoving it back in my pocket.

Quick change. I smile at them, her sitting on the bed, fully dressed, him squeezed in to one of our lesser armchairs. Dorothy's husband intrigues me. He visited her almost every day, but rarely talks, and unlike Sheila's brother-in-law, who seems to be silent because he's angry and scared, Dorothy's husband comes across as simply not in the habit of talking. Maybe she does the talking for both of them. He's short and big-bellied and his hips bulge out slightly under the chair's stiff wooden arms. Maybe that's why he's so quiet. Maybe he doesn't want to complain about his uncomfortable chair.

"I'm sorry about the wait. A little too much going on at once today, but now I'm ready, so let's get you out of here. You've got how long of a drive home?" I'm talking too fast, trying to drown out any irritation they have.

"It's two hours," Dorothy says. "But he—" she gestures toward her husband, "he hates driving after dark so he wants to leave as soon as we can." Her eyes shift from him back to me and I see that she's frustrated with him, not with me, which is unfortunate, but I'm just relieved I won't have to apologize for eating lunch.

"This is for you." I hand her the special envelope. "And we can go through everything together, because I've got a copy also." I brandish it as proof.

She looks at the envelope, peers inside, then pulls out the stapled set of papers. "Mmm—umhmm—" she nods, "and there's my Prilosec," she says, looking up to quickly meet my eyes before she continues reading.

"The next two pages tell you when to take each medication, morning, noon, or night, and what the dose is."

"Uh-huh," she's not really listening, but I keep talking anyway.

"And—" my phone rings.

Dorothy keeps reading. "Oh, you can get that."

I click my phone to answer it and hear: "This is escort. I'm here for Moore. Um, could you come out in the hallway for a minute? We have a problem."

Only a door separates me from the caller, but the distance feels huge. Staying in the room will allow me to discharge Dorothy, and that will be the only thing I have to focus on for as long as it takes to get her out of the hospital. Leaving the room will cause more delay since who knows what I'm needed for or how long whatever it is may take.

"I actually need you, her nurse, I think," the escort says into the phone and I hear Candace's voice in the background: "I'm not doing that. I'm not doing that without an explanation!"

"I'll be right out." Clicking off the phone I look up at Dorothy. "Hey, I'll be right back. Just need to sort out something in the hallway."

"Oh, it's fine," Dorothy says, carefully reading through the packet of papers I gave her. I see her husband slightly roll his eyes and quietly sigh. He wants to drive home in daylight, but I have to do my job for Dorothy and Candace. Let's see if I can satisfy everyone.

Passing through the doorway I step into an argument. Candace confronts me. "She," she gestures toward the escort worker, "says I have to go on the stretcher, but no one told me that before."

"No one told you that on other visits to the hospital?"

"No. No one told me that *now*, this time, about this test."

I'm not understanding. "Is there something wrong with the stretcher?" I ask her.

"No. But no one told me I have to sit on it and now she's telling me I have to." The escort, who is turned away from Candace, holds up her hands in a gesture of helplessness. I look at her inquiringly, when suddenly I get it.

"I'm sorry no one told you about the stretcher." I keep my voice even. After all, this is about control. "They insist on it at CT, even for healthy patients like you." I use air quotes around "healthy" so it won't offend her. "Even for something as straightforward"—I stop myself from saying "simple"—"as checking a line. Do you mind going on the stretcher?"

"I don't mind at all," she's suddenly much calmer. "It's just that no one told me."

"Right. Well, thanks for being accommodating. You know, you could even walk to CT next to the stretcher if I say it's OK. They just want a stretcher there with you."

"No, I can go on the stretcher. See?" She stands with her back to it and with a hop settles herself onto it, then gracefully swivels her legs to lie down. "Wait. I need my phone," she hops back off the stretcher and walks back into her room to get it.

Score another one for empathy. *Thank you*, I mouth to the escort. "I'll see you when she's done."

I can tell that stubborn wrinkle is there between my eyebrows. I just want to finish with Dorothy—it shouldn't be so hard.

One time I created a time-free bubble for myself to focus exclusively on a discharge. I could call it a gift to my young patient, but it was a gift for me as well. Work had felt high pressure and scattered for weeks. I wanted to experience really doing something right.

The patient, Jenn, was in her early twenties. She deserved to have things done right, too. Her diagnosis of leukemia came out of the blue, as it does for everyone, but she'd only recently moved to Pittsburgh after getting married. Except for her new husband she was alone in the city.

She was one of those rare people who was filled with goodwill. In a fairy tale, flowers would have bloomed behind her as she walked. Her newly bald head covered with a cheap bandanna, she never betrayed any bitterness about the poor timing of her disease. I sometimes wondered if all that generosity of spirit was real, if anyone could be so consistently nice. She must have had selfish, lonely moments, but we never saw them in the hospital.

The day I discharged her Lucy was her nurse practitioner. Jenn didn't have a lot of money and there were insurance issues, so the supplies she needed at home wouldn't show up on time. Lucy asked me to load Jenn up with saline flushes and latex gloves and to show her how to care for her central line since, like Candace, she would go home with it remaining in place on her chest.

In our supply room I grabbed wrapped saline syringes, a box of alcohol wipes, and gloves in her size. Technically I was stealing from the hospital, but nurses do it when it's either pilfer or leave the patient without proper care at home. The real cost of the supplies was negligible.

I brought my phone into Jenn's room, but told myself I wouldn't answer it if it rang while I was discharging her. I also moved the usual set of concerns—an antibiotic to be hung, a phone call to return, a tube of blood to draw and send to the lab—to the back of my mind. *For as long as it takes*, I thought, *I'm talking to her.*

The paperwork was quick. She had learned well during her six-week crash course in leukemia. The hard part would be taking care of her central line. It makes people understandably nervous to go home with a piece of medical hardware hanging out of their body. Jenn had the typical Hickman catheter with three separate tubes, or lumens, hanging down from the insertion site on her upper chest. Each of those tubes needed to be injected with saline every day and each day Jenn also needed to verify that blood could be pulled from each one. To me it's mindless work because I've done it so many times, but I might be worried if I had to care for my own line myself. Jenn had learned about her IV line amid the flurry of treatment and the doldrums of count recovery.

Sitting in a chair across from her while she sat on the bed, I explained the process and that it had to be done every day. The lumens are color-coded red, white, and blue, and I advised her to do them in that order so she wouldn't skip one accidentally. I picked up the red lumen, scrubbed the top of it for fifteen seconds with an alcohol wipe, then screwed a syringe of saline onto the red lumen and pushed the plunger in. It slid in easily.

"This is the flush," I told her, "and then you stop, pull back on the plunger like this." I held the syringe with my left hand and drew back with my right until the expected thin stream of blood swirled into the saline. "That's your blood return. That lets you know the line is working and in the right place."

She watched me carefully. I did the white lumen and had her do the blue to show me that she knew how. She hesitated when twisting on the saline flush and pushing in the plunger, but when she pulled back, drawing a rush of blood into the syringe, she smiled without reservation. Then, like I'd shown her, she pushed in the whole 10 ml of saline, unscrewed the syringe, and re-closed the clamp lock on the line.

"See. Piece of cake." She laughed.

"I wrote the steps down here," I handed her a piece of paper. "Read them and see if they make sense."

She read through the instructions, keeping her head very still, and when she was done, nodded solemnly.

"You've got this!" I said, and we hugged, teacher and student, very pleased with her success. Last, I showed her the items I'd packed up and put all of them into a bigger plastic bag.

And maybe there is some cosmic force for justice, at least in small things, because my phone didn't ring and I didn't think about anything but her discharge during the twenty-five minutes I stayed in her room.

> Man was made for Joy and Woe
> And when this we rightly know
> Thro' the World we safely go

William Blake's poem again finds wisdom in a simple truth: "Some to Misery are born" while others "are Born to sweet delight." Jenn embodied both possibilities. She was a joy of a human being who'd been struck with a woeful disease; the sustaining love she felt from her husband offered delight amid her misery. I like to think that by giving her so much focused attention on the day of her discharge I contributed to her ability to travel safely through the world.

Remembering my time with Jenn, I close my ears and eyes to any other needs when I return to Dorothy's room. It looks as if neither she nor her husband has moved, but there are now two suitcases resting against the bed and I see that all the photographs are gone from her walls. "We're ready to go," she says, a funny kind of Mary Poppins hat on her head and a dark wool coat lying next to her.

"Great. I just need you to sign here," I tell her, flipping to the correct page and pointing at the signature line.

"Looks like you'll need a wheelchair for yourself and one for everything you brought," I say, looking at the two suitcases, the purple comforter folded on the bed, the jigsaw puzzle on the table in its box.

"That's right. And he can push one of them." She gestures again toward her husband. "I'll hold the comforter. The puzzle can go in this bag and hang off a handle on the wheelchair." This is how Dorothy likes it to be, I realize. Despite how agreeable she usually was at the hospital, she wants to be in charge, and that includes packing.

"I'll call escort for the wheelchairs—" but before I even press any numbers on the phone, it rings.

I hear the polite and quiet voice of the escort, "Could you come out here one more time?"

"Right *now*?" I ask. Can't I just finish this? Can't I just get Dorothy out of here?

I hear Candace's sharp voice over the phone.

"I'm coming."

"Calling for the wheelchairs *right now*," I tell Dorothy, holding up the phone and dialing ostentatiously while I open the door to her room and go out.

Candace starts to talk, then sees me on the phone. Her eyes get small and the skin around her mouth pinches at her lips. Smiling, I hold up a hand, hoping it communicates "please wait, I'll be right with you," rather than, "dear God, what is it now?"

I put in my order for two wheelchairs, then hang up and look at Candace.

"I'm ready. I just thought you'd be here when I left. After I got my phone from my room, you were gone." Her voice is acid; it stings. But underneath I hear something else—hurt. And then Candace's full history comes back to me. I first met Candace a few months ago and she told me about her serious surgery from a few years earlier where everything went horribly wrong. It wasn't our hospital and I didn't know the docs. She was scarred, literally, with a jagged criss-cross on her lower abdomen. She showed it to me. It took months before the pain completely went away and though she hadn't wanted children, she would no longer be able to have them after that operation.

I had forgotten all of that, and remembering now, I look at her, try to really see her, all of her, not just the upward jerk of her chin, the accusatory voice. "I'm so sorry. Got caught up."

"I just thought you'd be here. That's all. It doesn't matter," she says, turning away from me and hopping up on the stretcher again.

"You're right; I didn't explain. I'll see you when you get back." She ignores me and the escort looks at me, grimaces sympathetically, then starts to push the carriage down the hall. I feel bereft, for a second, but then I hear the chime of a call bell and see that Sheila's light is on. Dammit! She must need more pain medicine and Dorothy isn't yet out of here.

I turn toward Dorothy's room and my phone rings. What now? I'm drowning in details, moving as fast as I can, but in truth not moving at all. Giving Dorothy that final push home depends on me. Getting Sheila to the OR, safely, depends on me. Hooking Mr. Hampton up to his drug depends on me, as does making sure it doesn't kill him. And Candace; caring for her without saying something I regret, or in my distraction missing a detail that makes all the difference, also depends on me.

My hands feel tingly, my throat tight. It's the beginning of panic. I only have four patients. Four. How can taking care of them feel so impossible?

I USED TO LOVE A comic book series called the *Legion of Super Heroes*. One of the super heroes, named Duo Damsel, often comes to mind when I'm at work. She could divide into two fully intact versions of herself just by concentrating. Maybe I could do that, too, if I tried really hard. Maybe just today—just this one time. If I really wanted it.

My phone keeps ringing. No matter how hard I concentrate, it'll only be me here. I hit the talk button. "Medical Oncology, Theresa." It's the OR scheduler. Sheila's set for 7 p.m. at the earliest. They couldn't get her in any sooner. "We need the pre-op checklist done *before* she gets here," the guy tells me.

Love the emphasis on *before*, as if I don't understand that "pre-op" indicates "prior to the operation." I want to respond with something clever or sarcastic, but I just say yes and hang up. What's the point? He may be a rude SOB, or maybe he's overworked like the rest of us, or both. I write down the OR time and then banish him from my memory.

Jesus! Call lights escalate in volume and frequency as time goes by and Sheila's now achieves the pitch of a warning in a bad action movie. Warning: the perimeter has been compromised!

I push hard on her door. "Sorry, sorry, sorry. Too much to do." Her face is a mask of deep lines and she's bent over in bed, her breath coming short and fast.

I reach behind her to turn off the chiming light. "Pain?" She nods and gulps. "I'll be right back with more medicine. And, hey," I move my eyes around the room, connect with her sister and brother-in-law, "the OR has you scheduled for seven tonight so that's our ballpark." Her sister sits next to Sheila, holding her hand. The husband is standing up beside her, his hands stuck tight in his front jeans pockets.

"Seven," he says, and nods, just once.

"I'll be right back." Down the hall, into the locked drug room, pulling up Sheila's record on the locked narcotics machine, picking the drug, double-checking the dose, counting the number of syringes already in the drawer, and entering that number into the computer. It says my count is wrong. I recount and get the same number. Again it says my count is wrong. "Fuck it." I hit the button to go ahead and pull out one pre-filled syringe. So there'll be a discrepancy. I'm not fixing it now.

Around the corner and up the hall I go as fast as I can without running. Screw a needle onto an empty syringe, alcohol the top of the narcotic tube, then pull out the Dilaudid and squirt it into 10 ml of saline. Sheila's lined face is all I see; I hear her stabbing breath. The pain got ahead of her.

Back into her room and I pivot so fast from my medcart that my shoes squeak on the floor. I hold up the syringe, show it to her, then pick up her running IV and inject the drug into the line after first wiping it with alcohol. Then I wipe it again and push in another 10 ml of saline, to make sure the narcotic gets into her bloodstream fast.

She sighs and closes her eyes, then leans back against the pillow at the head of the bed. "Thank you," her sister says, and her voice, quiet in the dark room, quavers. The husband nods again then sits back down in the embracing armchair.

"I paged a minister for you. I don't—I don't know when she'll get here." Then I leave them; I don't even look to make sure they heard.

I should also re-check Sheila's blood pressure, but I'll give the Dilaudid fifteen minutes or so and then go back in.

While I chart Sheila's drug on the computer along with the multi-step "pain assessment," I look at Candace's open door and, somewhat unkindly, hope she has a very long wait once she gets to interventional radiology.

Suddenly our other clinician, the half-bedside nurse/half-management partner to Nancy the charge-nurse, finds me at my medcart. "I just got back from my meetings. Sounds like you're having a day." Her name is Marilyn and she's got the most beautiful green eyes as well as a preternatural calm. "What can I do for you?"

"Can you give Mr. Hampton his pre-meds for Rituxan? We need to get that started ASAP."

"Sure!" she says.

I pop into Dorothy's room. "The wheelchairs are coming. Do you need any help getting ready to go?"

"No. We're all ready. It's just—" she inclines her head to me, hinting there's something she wants to conspire about. I bend down and she starts to speak quietly. "Now, I took my candy dish, but I left you the candy. It's all here." She pulls out the top drawer of her nightstand and I see bags full of brightly colored paper, all in patterns familiar to me from my own childhood: mini Snickers, tiny Reese's Peanut Butter Cups, and Hershey's Kisses. "I don't want it to be forgotten."

"We don't want it to be forgotten, either, Dorothy. I'll put it in the break room right now." I pick up the plastic bags and cradle them like a baby. Turning, I see her husband smile. His mouth forms a slim rectangle, but the outer edges turn up just enough that it has to be a smile. "Thanks for this! The wheelchairs should be here soon!" I say, heading off to our conference room with my spoils.

I dump the bags of candy on the conference table and the silver and gold foil wrappers twinkle at me. Just one. I slip a Snickers in my pocket, hover over a Hershey's Kiss, leave it. Sheila's blood pressure!

I run into Marilyn on my way back to my medcart. She whispers to me. "Theresa, when you asked me to pre-med your guy for Rituxan you didn't tell me he was already half-dead."

"Yeah, I told them that. We're all a little concerned." I say, shaking my head.

"Well, he's ready to go and I charted the meds." She smiles at me.

"You so rock! Thank you!"

"You'll get my bill. Gotta go help Susie now."

She walks up the hall, passing a tall attractive man who stops when he approaches me and extends his hand. "Hi!" he says, "I'm Trace Hampton, Richard Hampton's son. Are you Theresa?"

"Yes. Hi!" I say, surprised at how movie-star handsome he is, with high cheekbones and thick brushed-back hair.

"I'm a little bit late," he says easily.

I check my watch: 3:30 pm. "Oh no, it's fine. He just got his pre-meds. I've, um, had a busy day."

"Well, then we're both on time." His smile is welcoming,

his voice relaxed. I look for a resemblance to his frail father, but except for the height, see none. "A friend of mine's coming, too," he says, "Stephen. If you can direct him in . . ." He gestures toward his dad's room.

"Sure," I tell him. "Stephen." He keeps standing next to me, as if he wants to say more, when two escorts arrive with their two wheelchairs for Dorothy and her paraphernalia. "Sorry. I've got to get a patient out of here."

"Oh, of course," He's so gracious. The tightness in my throat, the tension in my arms that came when I so much wanted to split in two, releases just a little.

There's a bustle outside Dorothy's room as the escort moves in both wheelchairs. I'm going to help, when I see Peter coming down the hall toward Sheila's room. I'm surprised by the look on his face. He's angry. I've never seen him angry. He's holding papers in his hands. He must be here to have Sheila sign the consent forms for her surgery.

What a mess this whole thing was from the start, I realize. They should have scanned her abdomen last night at 3 a.m. when she first showed up in the emergency department. Then the Argatroban might never have been started and she might have already been operated on.

Now, though, Peter will operate into the night, even though a tired doc, or nurse, is just as impaired as a tired truck driver or airline pilot. Work hours are limited for resident physicians, but why the workload for all MDs isn't regulated as carefully as some other professions is unclear. Is it because doctors' mistakes due to exhaustion only have the potential to kill one person, not many? Or perhaps as a culture we want to believe that physicians are superhuman, and some docs want to believe that of themselves.

Problem is they're not; no one is. Peter at least is smart enough to know he has limits, but on the other hand, time is working against us here. In the hospital we say "Time is muscle" for heart attack victims and "Time is brain" for stroke patients, indicating that the sooner those patients get the care they need the less heart or brain damage they will have. In Sheila's case, the bacteria will reproduce exponentially in her abdomen as time passes, and more of her intestine may die. The longer we wait the sicker she potentially becomes.

I want to go into Sheila's room, be there when she signs the consent, make sure she understands, check her blood pressure, but Dorothy's on her way out of the hospital.

"Are you her nurse? I'm gonna need some help stacking these belongings." The escort is new, learning the job. Helping with discharge is one of the things we get evaluated on when patients answer surveys about the quality of their care.

Dorothy's room is right next to Sheila's, but I walk into Dorothy's and Peter walks into Sheila's and we don't even say hello.

"OK, let's get you out of here, Dorothy."

We get the suitcases on one wheelchair, Dorothy in the other. She insists on loading everything in a precise way, but eventually it gets done and her belongings appear well-arranged. As she settles herself down I check the closet and the bathroom one last time, peak at the space under the bed. The card table was ours, not hers. It will need to be scrubbed down with anti-bacterial wipes, but I can leave that to housekeeping, I think. The rules about who cleans up what after a discharge occasionally change.

The husband raises himself from his confining chair, gives his large glasses a slight adjustment, and walks to the wheel-chair holding Dorothy. He grasps the handles and looks straight ahead, out the door of Dorothy's room.

"You make sure to share that candy," Dorothy bends around to tell me, arms encircling the purple comforter on her lap.

"I don't know, Dorothy. Maybe after I pick out the Hershey's Kisses for myself."

She laughs at the same time as Peter comes out of Sheila's room. He doesn't stop, just keeps walking up the hall. My throat feels tight again. How long has it been since I checked Sheila's blood pressure? I don't look at my watch; the time itself doesn't matter, but I need to do it soon and make sure that last shot of Dilaudid helped.

"Good-bye everyone," Dorothy calls out as she rolls down the hall. She waves with her right hand cupped, fingers together like a queen. Then she giggles as she blows kisses. No matter what happens today, I will make sure to remember this moment. When we've made you better, there's nothing as satisfying as leaving the hospital.

CHAPTER 9

Judgment Calls

Hey, sorry I couldn't be in here when the surgeon got your consent for the operation." I head right to Sheila, wrap the blood pressure cuff around her left arm, and pump up the balloon. The whole family looks as if the last bit of life energy they had just got wrung out of them. I need to know what Peter said.

The IV pump beeps as the cuff tightens, cutting off the flow of fluid up Sheila's arm. I silence it, then listen through my stethoscope for the tell-tale clicks that register her pressure: 152 is the first click and silence comes after 90. It's the sound of blood flowing through thousands of miles of arteries and veins pumped by a heart that never rests.

I let the pressure in the cuff fully run out and hear the Velcro rip as I take the cuff off Sheila's arm. I've done this so many times, yet it always feels like insight gained from a look inside a patient's body. Two numbers tell me if all is well or if something is starting to go very wrong.

The first few times those numbers were wrong came as a shock. Not shock from concern over my patient, though I felt that, too, but steeped as I was in the study of literature, I wasn't used to the idea that events in books, even if they're textbooks, can become real.

"Can you double-check a pressure for me?" I asked Gloria, the friend who teased me today about my yogurt spoon. She was about to say no, that she didn't have time, but there must have been something about the look on my face that made her change her mind.

She took the patient's pressure, looked up at me, eyes narrowed and firm. "Sixty over thirty."

"I got seventy over forty." We spoke quietly, looking right at each other. I'd read about severe hypotension, seen it before, but I was still a new enough nurse that the reality of detecting it surprised me. The patient had grown increasingly confused during the day and now was only semi-conscious. Those symptoms probably arose from the drug he was on, called Interleukin-2, but his drop in blood pressure would only make them worse.

"You OK?" Gloria asked me, using our shorthand for "Do you need help?" and if so, what should she do?

"No. I think I'm OK. I'll page the resident."

She called back right away. Everyone is on high alert when patients get IL-2. "I'll be right there. At that level I'm worried his organs won't be fully perfused."

She spelled it out like that, as if she, like me, was remembering her textbook. Perfusion: the nub of life is red blood cells oxygenating every part of our bodies.

The patient went to the ICU and they put him on vasopressors, drugs that raise blood pressure and keep it at a healthy level. He came back to us the next day, restored fully to himself, though with very little memory of the last twenty-four hours.

"You lived to tell the tale," I said, which seemed to make him feel better, even courageous. At least he knew there was a story to be told.

But Sheila's blood pressure is holding steady now. "One fifty-two over ninety. Like usual, you're a little high, which for now is good." I tell Sheila, looking at the IV tubing and eyeing the amount of fluid left in the bag. Then I realize Sheila and her family aren't hearing a word I say; what did Peter say when I couldn't be in the room?

Sheila's sister purses her lips, gestures at the door. "He said," she pauses and blinks a few times, "he said they might wait until tomorrow to operate."

"What?" I blurt out.

Sheila, sunk back once again under a pile of blankets, seems to be melting like a lump of wax into an amalgamation of pain, confusion, and hopelessness.

"Let me talk to him. I'll go now and try to catch him." Hurry. Out the door, up the hallway. I must ask Peter why and then tell him that the idea of waiting another day for surgery seems inexplicable and terrifying to Sheila.

I'm lucky. He's heading out the door, toward the elevators, when I call out.

"Theresa, you just can't stop bothering Dr. Coyne, can you?" our secretary calls out, loud enough for anyone standing nearby to hear. This is a moment when I find her effusiveness difficult.

I try to ignore her, but then I feel it: upset. The secretary's comment suggests I'm not adhering to the expected MD-RN relationship. I feel exposed, and it's not the first time, as an opinionated, even a pushy nurse. But why is that? Shouldn't I feel assertive and responsible, instead? Aren't those core values for all health-care professionals?

The two best articles I've read on how physicians and nurses work together are called "The Doctor-Nurse Game" and "The Doctor-Nurse Game Revisited," both by Leonard I. Stein, a psychiatrist. The first article came out in 1967, the second in 1990. There is no data in these articles, no carefully tabulated results from original research, but the sting of painful truths comes through.

The word "game" itself refers not to child's play, but to psychologically intricate interactions governed by rules, even if the rules are not consciously acknowledged. The MD-RN relationship is historically rooted in gender differences and the condescension and imperiousness that marked men's relationships with women a century ago. Many women have now become doctors and men are increasingly becoming nurses, but vestiges of the history remain.

In the sixties Dr. Stein wrote that if a nurse had an idea about patient care, the unwritten rules of the Doctor-Nurse game dictated that her recommendations appear to be the doctor's ideas all along. The nurse might say, when discussing a patient with insomnia: "Pentobarbital mg 100 was quite effective night before last," and the doctor would relay back to her, "Pentobarbital mg 100 before bedtime as needed for sleep, got it?" The drug and dose are the nurse's ideas, but the MD is allowed to rephrase them as his own.

Dr. Stein revisited the doctor-nurse game in 1990, and this time he described the nurse as a "stubborn rebel." Rather than giving the doctor a clinical script, the nurse cast herself as a corrective agent to the doctor's potential incompetence. The pentobarbital scenario becomes a confrontation instead of a polite, carefully calibrated exchange: "Mrs. Jones can't sleep. She needs pentobarbital." The nurse would probably be figured standing with her hands on her hips, head thrust forward, and implicit in her tone would be the unspoken challenge, "Your patient's in need; what are you gonna do about it?"

There are nurses who hate these articles and I understand why—neither image of our profession is flattering. But I know I have played both these games and all possible permutations in between. Hospital nurses get hired and fired independent of MDs, but from what I see and hear, at a fair number of hospitals no nurse would be protected if an important doctor really wanted her gone. Doctors are our shadow bosses, the people whose orders we put into action, whose patients we share the care of, even though the MDs don't explicitly supervise us. No wonder we both end up playing games when we communicate at work.

But Peter's not like that. Now he stops immediately, ready to listen. I put the secretary's words out of my mind, try not to think about whether anyone is watching me with a critical eye. "Sheila said you may wait until tomorrow to operate." He nods. He doesn't look angry anymore, just as if he also resents the impossibility of being two places at once.

"If you could operate tonight, that would be so much better for her. I know anesthesia needs to prep her and that regardless, you could get that out of the way tonight, but with the amount of pain she's in I hate for her to go down, meet with anesthesia, come back up to the floor, and then go back down to the OR again tomorrow morning."

"It may be better to wait until tomorrow." He hears me, but he's looking out the door toward the elevators.

I'm not sure what to say. He's the surgeon; the decision about whether to operate has to be his. It won't be my hand holding the knife. There must be a weighing of how dire Sheila's situation is and how tired he and the rest of his team will be. I know from experience that fatigue is a thief of concentration and memory because I lived it when my twins were babies. Peter, I'm sure, also knows how dangerous fatigue is.

When doctors and nurses train, the idea is to push through exhaustion, ignore it, transcend it, but only the rarest of us can really do that without drugs to help, and no one, even with chemical stimulants, can do it forever. Humans need sleep as much as we need food and water, and when we don't get enough our minds fray at the edges. Sleep is said to clean our brains; tired people can make mistakes without even realizing what they're doing. Shakespeare knew it: "Sleep knits up the raveled sleeve of care." This is poetry and truth. It may be better to wait until tomorrow, Peter said. He could be right. A decision like this is all about weighing the risks and benefits. Only he knows how tired he is, how much the week has already worn on him, what else he has to accomplish this day.

But what about Sheila? Overnight the bacteria will proliferate inside her abdomen and parts of her colon that aren't now dead may begin to die, or will finish dying. That is also truth. Tissue damage at that level can't be repaired; it has to be cut out by the, perhaps exhausted, surgeon. The multiplying bacteria will have to be killed by large doses of intravenous antibiotics. The longer Sheila waits with her gut oozing inside her own body, the closer she gets to a point of no return.

No surgical protocol or clinical algorithm will make clear in advance what the best timing is for her specific case. For one patient the wait won't matter. For another it could be the difference between living and dying. For one surgeon the fatigue won't overcome years of training and professional discipline. For another it could be the moment when he hits the wall of his own vulnerability. No crystal ball exists to reveal which patient and surgeon we have today.

I, the nurse, am here for Sheila, who's worried and in pain. Peter's my friend and colleague, but Sheila's my responsibility, so I make my request one more time. "If tonight works." Pushy or patient advocate? He nods his head just slightly then turns to the elevators he's been eyeing and before I can say "Thanks for thinking about it," he's gone.

Dave the pharmacy tech walks up behind me with the

Rituxan for Mr. Hampton. He's got a low deep voice, almost a growl, but he's often quite funny and his eyes crinkle up when he laughs. "Rituxan for Richard Hampton." He hands me the bag full of clear liquid.

This is the next-to-last step of chemotherapy administration. The process started when Mr. Hampton's attending physician decided to give him Rituxan. Then the pregnant oncology fellow wrote the order and brought it over to me so that I could double-check it with another nurse. Afterwards I left the verified order for pharmacy and they took the order and mixed the drug according to specifications. Finally Dave delivered the drug to me and all I have to do now is set it up to intravenously infuse into Mr. Hampton.

It's a complicated and well-rehearsed protocol because chemotherapy, like surgery, almost always comes with Faustian trade-offs. We kill your cancer but your hair falls out, you have unrelenting diarrhea, permanent nerve pain and/or mouth sores so bad you can't eat. Rituxan is different in that it mobilizes the patient's own immune system to attack the disease. Since the rare person can die from a bee sting or eating a peanut— the result of an extreme overreaction of the immune system—it's difficult to predict what will happen when a patient receives a drug like Rituxan, and the trouble it brings usually happens during the infusion: a precipitous drop in blood pressure, shaking that can't be controlled, a racing heart, severe shortness of breath.

I check my watch. How did it get to be 4:30 p.m.? Well,

at least the passing of time ensures the pre-meds that Marilyn gave are definitely active in Mr. Hampton's body so I can connect the Rituxan to his IV.

"Theresa!" It's Nora and Amy, who helped me by taking lunch to Susie's patient. "Want some?" says Amy, holding up a gift card to the coffee shop across the street.

"Oh my God, you are lifesavers! Where did you get that? And how do you have time?"

"We-ell," Amy says, "Remember the Vaughans?"

I nod. "Oh gosh, they were so-o-o-o nice."

"Yeah, well, he had an outpatient appointment in the clinic and they came and dropped this off." There's probably some rule about how we're not supposed to accept gifts from patients if they are connected to a cash amount, but I've never heard of it being enforced.

"So how do you have time to do this?"

"We don't," Amy says, "but we both really need some caffeine and it's free!"

I lower my voice and look at Nora, "How's Mr. King in the ICU?"

She shrugs one shoulder, looks away, then shakes her head.

"Medium skim latte?" Amy asks me brightly. She's writing down orders on a notecard.

"You know me well. Thanks." I'm suddenly overjoyed. Is this how addicts feel before getting a fix? Oh, who cares—even if I am a junkie, it's only espresso and milk.

Back at my medcart I think of Sheila and her family. I feel

the weight of the Rituxan—it's almost a half-liter and has some heft—in my hand then set it down on my medcart. I need to tell Sheila and her family what Peter said, but I'm so tired of hurry up and wait for this kind and fragile woman and I dread confirming the uncertainty about when the operation will be.

Remember. I make myself remember that she could be my sister, my mother, me. I would want to know what the surgeon said. I would want a nurse who told me what was up as soon as she knew. I try to summon courage, fortitude from wherever they are in my body, pull it up to my brain from my toes.

It's quiet where I stand. I turn back to my medcart, pick up the Rituxan. I could hang it and then talk to Sheila and her family. It would take fifteen, twenty minutes to check the drug, grab some vitals, hook it up, and record all that on the computer. Dorothy's gone, Candace is off the floor, and Irving's yet to arrive. I could get the Rituxan going—making things a little easier for night shift since the sooner the drug starts the sooner it, and all the checks it requires, are done—then tell Sheila what's going on.

But I don't.

I go into the dark room. Sheila and her family have never raised the blinds. Perhaps the sunlight would have been another unwelcome sensory experience, or maybe they just never thought of opening them. I could have offered, except that right now evening is coming and the sun will soon set anyway.

They all look up expectantly as soon as I walk in and I know then it was right to come in here before hanging the Rituxan. "Hey, I just talked to Peter Coyne. He's going to try for tonight."

The sister raises her head to me and her shoulders, tight and hunched forward, relax back into her chair as Sheila closes her eyes and the lines on her face, just for a moment, disappear, making her skin appear smooth. "It may not work, though. It may have to be tomorrow"—I improvise a little here— "depending on how your blood is clotting and what the schedule in the operating room is. I'll tell you as soon as I know anything."

I thought this information would deflate them all over again—I haven't told them much new—but it doesn't. They seem to understand that many factors influence when Peter will operate, not just timing or his own personal preference. They may have just wanted an acknowledgment that not knowing is hard, because when I finish talking they all nod, the brother-in-law's chin doing one slow up and down.

"I've got to start chemo in another room." I point my thumb backward at the door. "Can I get you anything?" Sheila's brother-in-law gives a shake of the head no and her sister breathes out and settles back into her chair. Ambiguity is anxiety-producing, but the appearance of indifference combined with a lack of control may be what mattered the most here.

John Keats, the nineteenth-century poet, recognized the challenges posed by lack of hard knowledge and the strength it takes to endure in such situations by coining the term "Negative Capability," which he defined as: "when a man is capable of being in uncertainties, mysteries, doubts, without any irritable reaching after fact and reason." Keats spent his adult life fighting tuberculosis and died at age twenty-five, so for him the "irritable reaching after fact" was not merely poetic or theoretical. He knew what would kill him, and soon—"for many a time / I have been half in love with easeful Death"—and yet his art triumphed over his affliction.

Out in the hallway I close my eyes briefly to clear my head and Marilyn, like an apparition of helpfulness, appears at my shoulder. "Thought you might need a checker for the Rituxan."

"Thank you."

"Brought you this, too," she says, handing me a thick blue plastic gown.

"You are the greatest."

"And this." She holds up Mr. Hampton's chart.

"I could kiss you."

"Please don't."

"Here we go." Inside, Mr. Hampton's room is a different world from Sheila's. He's using the oxygen of course and he looks awfully pale, but no one in this room is at all worried. His son Trace and Trace's friend are in the room and all three of them look as relaxed as if this is just an ordinary day.

Trace waves to Marilyn and me, an easy, friendly movement of his hand, then gestures to the man sitting beside him. "This is Stephen," he says, like a seasoned host introducing friends at a cocktail party.

Mr. Hampton even waves at us and I reach forward to pick up his wrist, read off his wrist band. Name. Birth date. Medical record number. Marilyn checks them against the same information on the chemotherapy order in his chart. Then I lay his wrist back down on the bed, but not before patting the back of his hand. When possible, touch in the hospital should come with a dose of kindness.

Marilyn holds up the Rituxan and reads off the information on the bag of drug. Patient name. Birth date. Medical Record Number. Drug. Dose. Rate of Administration. I double-check everything she reads against the chemotherapy order. It all checks. His base rate is 25 ml/hour and after one hour I'll turn it up to 50 ml/hour and leave it there. Jeez Louise. This bag will take all night to go in.

Marilyn pulls up Mr. Hampton's chart on the computer in the room and together we initial our double-check of the patient and the drug, referring back to the paper chart, too, but officially confirming everything in the computer.

Marilyn winks at me as she leaves, taking the chart with her. "I'm here if you need me," she says.

"This is when I get in costume," I tell them, pulling on a pair of chemo-protective gloves, then putting on the blue plastic gown that Marilyn brought me. I leave it open to the back with the tie doubled-around and knotted in front and pull on another set of gloves, making sure the glove ends cover the soft white cuffs on the chemo gown, protecting the skin on my wrists.

I hook up a liter bag of saline as a "just in case," as in, just in case his blood pressure severely drops I can turn off the Rituxan and load him up with fluid quickly from the big bag of normal saline. Giving lots of liquid fast is the standard first-line response to hypotension.

I pick up one lumen of Mr. Hampton's PICC line from his

upper arm and connect the saline to it, checking first for the flash of blood in the line. Then I connect the Rituxan to the line of saline. "This is the drug," I point to the Rituxan, "and this is just saline. He's only getting the one smaller bag."

This is modern medicine: a plastic bag of what looks like water contains one of the best drugs we have against lymphoma.

I now insert the clamp on the Rituxan tubing and the section of tubing immediately after it into the IV pump. I unclamp the tubing, unroll the roller clamp farther down the line, and start the pump, which makes a soft purring noise as I look at the drip chamber just below the bag and see one clear drop form and fall.

My orders say I need to take vital signs every fifteen minutes for the first hour and it's a good idea since Mr. Hampton is so fragile. I will be in and out of his room for the next hour, checking and watching.

I pull off my first layer of gloves and gown, then the second layer, wad them up together, and throw them away in the hard yellow plastic chemo waste bin in Mr. Hampton's room. It's not that coming in contact with Rituxan by itself is so toxic, but for nurses who give chemotherapy, repeat "unintentional exposure" to biohazards from spills, accidental contact, or drugs that aerosolize, could threaten our health. When working with chemo we take a "better safe than sorry" approach. Pregnant nurses never even hang chemo. Why take the risk?

"I think you've already heard about this drug, but let me tell you about it one more time." Trace and his friend Stephen incline their torsos forward just a little bit, listening. "Rituxan can be a tough drug. A lot of people get it and do just fine. Some people, though, have a really bad reaction to it: hives, itching, shortness of breath, rigors—uncontrollable shaking—fever, sudden sweats, an overall feeling of yuck!" They laugh. They like the description "yuck!" "So, if he feels in any way unusual, put on the call light immediately and get me in here, OK?" I point to the nurse button on the TV remote and behind the bed. "I'd rather you call me in for nothing than wait and have things get pretty bad."

The two of them nod energetically. "I'll be back in . . ." I look at my watch, "ten minutes." Before I go out the door I give Mr. Hampton a quick look. He remains supine in bed but his eyes are wide open and bright. Well, the drug's started. I'll monitor him and keep on my toes.

Outside in the hallway my phone rings. It's the interventional radiologist; the doc who did the dye study on Candace's central line. "Her line's completely fine," he announces. "In fact, she couldn't even tell me what was wrong with it." I'm not sure what I can say since I didn't order the study and received no extra information about it beyond what Candace told me and what the order itself said: "Consult Interventional Radiology: STAT dye study of central line."

The IR physician keeps talking. "We put off other patients who really needed scans and stayed around later than usual to do this today all because of a STAT dye study. It's not really appropriate to put in a dye study STAT for a line that doesn't have an obvious problem."

Now I get it. He's annoyed with the oncologist who ordered

the scan for STAT—NOW—making him do this job when sicker patients possibly more in need could have gone first. I want to say, "Am I a doctor? Did I enter that order?" but I don't. It won't help. Nurses sometimes serve as intermediaries in this way: physicians take their frustrations with each other out on the bedside nurse because we're safer.

"This is . . . a very insistent patient," I say, trying to be diplomatic.

"Yeah, I got that," he sighs. "But this study didn't need to be done. The line was absolutely fine and her X-ray last week showed that."

"She had an X-ray last week that showed the line works fine?"

"Uh-huh."

"I didn't know that." Silence. Again, I'm not sure what to say.

"So it didn't need to be done, or at least not today ahead of other people with real problems."

"I hear you," I say, and then I drop my professionalism and just talk, human to human. "Hey. I'm sorry you had to stay late, I'm sorry other patients got put off. It's one of those situations . . ." My voice trails off. I can't explain Candace with a few bland, ameliorative phrases.

"It's not your fault," he says, the hard edge suddenly gone from his voice. "We just, we had to postpone a test that was a lot more important for someone else. I don't like making people wait for nothing."

"Right. Well, thanks for doing her study first. She does need the transplant to save her life, if that gives the dye study any more urgency."

And then he laughs. Maybe he appreciates irony. "Good luck with her. I think you're gonna need it."

"Indeed." I hang up and check my watch. Time to get Mr. Hampton's vital signs, make sure he's not in his room gasping for breath, though with his son sitting next to him that's unlikely.

Suddenly Amy's back, holding a paper tray of coffee drinks in matching white cups. "Your latte," she says, setting it down on the medcart before moving on, her blond hair shiny in the hospital's bright lights.

I pick up the cup and take a careful sip. It's hot but not scalding, and the frothiness of the milk, the bitterness of the coffee, hit my mouth like a pleasure bomb. It's just past 5 p.m. Two and a half more hours and then I go home.

CHAPTER 10

Faith

I have ten minutes before my next set of vitals is due and I again cycle mentally through my list of preoccupations: Sheila shouldn't need pain meds, Candace is off the floor, and Irving isn't here yet. I head up the hall. I need to look at a different set of ecru walls and maybe Beth has heard from her daughter.

Rounding the corner to her medcart, I almost run into her. I'm distracted, but she's ecstatic. "My daughter emailed me and then I just talked to her on the phone," she says, holding up her cell phone in her right hand like it's a prize she's won. "I know we're not supposed to talk on our cell phones at work, but I thought this would be OK." She's smiling and that tightness in her face is gone.

My mental image of a crashing helicopter, of black smoke and ripping screams is, thank goodness, replaced by a woman in fatigues running through the dust churned up by helicopter blades. The dust dries out her mouth, stings her eyes, settles like a mist in her hair, but she's on the ground and no one shoots at her as she runs. She's safe.

"Right now I'm having a very good day," Beth says. "Yes, a very good day."

"That is so great." I'm smiling so hard my face starts to feel stiff. This is excellent news. Because Beth's daughters are twins, like mine, the loss of one might be irrecoverable for the other. That person has been with you, literally, since the very beginning of both your lives.

Having twins is what got me into nursing, so I think about the connection between twins and being a nurse a lot. I never expected twins. Never. But because I was bigger than normal and very nauseated at the start of my pregnancy I had an early ultrasound, at eight weeks. When the ultrasound tech showed me those two glowing white blobs on her screen, their nascent hearts beating, I felt reverent and afraid. Could I do this? Handle two new lives at once?

Thirty-four weeks later they arrived, babies fully formed: Miranda and Sophia, wonder and wisdom. Labor had started at four in the morning. After I got to the hospital and changed into a gown I stood in the bathroom, arms bent, palms against the wall, having a contraction that felt like it would rip my belly apart. *Oh my God, how will I survive this*, I wondered, but the labor was quick. After just three hours, out they came, four minutes apart: two little bald heads, four eyes and ears, two brains ready to learn about the world, two beating hearts.

I fell in love with the mess of it all: hugs and crying and baskets of laundry and early smiles and sleeplessness and the joys of motherhood, in stereo. Midwives managed my pregnancy and after Miranda and Sophia were born I decided I wanted to be a midwife, to trade the books and classrooms of a university for the controlled chaos of the maternity ward. Midwifery got me into nursing and once I learned more about being a bedside RN, I knew I had found my professional home. Bringing two lives into the world in one day is not a small thing. It gave me a taste for the life-and-death struggles that are our daily bread in the hospital.

Consider my friend Beth. She has two daughters, twins, and one grew up to be a soldier, risking her life in a foreign land for an unsure goal and little glory. The mom works as a nurse, keeping the home fires burning, and this afternoon she hears that daughter's voice at the other end of a cell phone connection, on the other side of the earth, and knows her little girl, her daughter's twin, is safe. A ripple of joy goes through the universe. It's what we live for.

"What will you do tonight?"

"You know, Theresa, I'm just happy right now, just very happy. So I'll finish the day and go home and just be . . . happy." I give her a hug. There's nothing I can add to that.

"Do you need any help? I suddenly feel like I have all the time in the world," Beth says.

"No, I'm good. I may end up calling a rapid response on this guy, and then I'll need your help."

She raises her eyebrows. "Well, you know where to find me," she says.

Back at my medcart I see Doris, the minister I paged for Sheila and her family. She's wearing a blue-patterned cotton cardigan over her gray shirt with white clerical collar and her middle-aged belly makes her look pleasingly soft and huggable. Her short wavy brown hair halos her round face, setting off a wide smile. Presbyterian? I think she's Presbyterian. Denomination doesn't usually come up in the hospital.

"Sorry it took me so long. Had a meeting. Places to go, people to see."

I tell her about Sheila, the sister and brother-in-law, her perforated bowel, and the twenty percent chance of death statistic. She breathes in. "They asked for me?"

I nod, "Uh-huh."

"OK." She nods back firmly and I realize that I trust her. If I thought I might be dead tomorrow I'm not sure whom I would want to talk to, but I don't think I'd turn Doris away.

She knocks gently on the door to Sheila's room and I step into Mr. Hampton's.

"How's he doing?" Trace and Stephen both nod enthusiastically. I get his vital signs: the blood pressure cuff, the stethoscope, the pulse ox monitor, and the thermometer. He's stable. By these measures he's even fine. I look at him, scrunching my eyebrows together and tilting my head to the side. "How're you feeling?" Mr. Hampton shrugs. "Any shortness of breath? Feel like your heart is racing? Dizziness?" He shakes his head, no. "Itching?" he shakes his head again. I tilt my head the other way, studying him.

"You haven't seen any problems?" I ask Trace and Stephen.

They shake their heads no. I purse my lips, shrug. "That's good! Let me know if anything changes."

One more set of fifteen-minute vitals to get, then it switches to every half hour. I could ask an aide to get them for me, but with this drug and this patient I want to take the vital signs and observe him myself. If I know exactly what's going on it gives me the illusion of control.

I start a note on the computer about beginning the Rituxan infusion, how Mr. Hampton is doing, that his son is in the room with him. In my note I write VSS: vital signs stable. Then I enter the vitals I have so far into the computer, listing the precise times I took them. I've been lucky today—I was able to take them on time. Otherwise I battle with my conscience about what to write down: the actual times I got the vitals, or when I was *supposed* to take them. It's another nursing no-win. We shouldn't lie when documenting, but there's the not-able-to-be-two-places-at-once problem, which can make accurate charting ethically complicated. If I falsify records in small ways I worry I will end up being too comfortable with the idea of little, victimless lies. I don't want to get used to fudging records even for something as relatively trivial as this.

I check the orders tab—nothing new—go to the task list and see . . . I forgot to fill out the computer form that says Dorothy is gone.

I already put the discharge paperwork in her chart, but with electronic charting completing paperwork only on actual paper is not enough. I type a short missive into the computer verifying that Dorothy left the hospital in a wheelchair and that she "communicated understanding" of her discharge instructions. Then I fill out the discharge/transfer form on the computer, certifying that she planned to leave in a private vehicle (versus an ambulance) accompanied by her husband and went to her own home. It feels like the apotheosis of CYA charting.

My phone rings. Nancy, the charge nurse, has an update on Irving. The ambulance already left, but she doesn't know when. I look at my watch. It's almost 5:30. Most likely I'll be settling in Irving while sending Sheila off to her surgery. We hold the infinity of our patients' lives in our hands and yet I cannot hold Irving and Sheila—one coming the other going—in my two hands at the same time, although I may have to.

"Does he have a fever, pain?"

"I don't know. That's all they told me. But, you know, there's a lot of construction out that way and it's rush hour. They'll be at least an hour." She hangs up. I look at the phone. It doesn't seem necessary to be quite so abrupt but the traffic information is helpful.

Hey, wait a minute. Nancy was going to leave early, right? Maybe she got delayed and is trying to rush out of here, which has to be frustrating. She's not easy to work with as charge nurse, but I feel a pinch of empathy for her.

Irving has an abscess on his backside; a "boil on his butt." If I weren't focused on the timing with Sheila I might laugh. It's not funny and I'm sure it hurts, but that's the kind of Missouri-Ozarks phrase my dad would use. He was also fond of the vivid "Don't get your bowels in an uproar" and the vulgar, "Just hold on to your pecker" if he thought someone was being impatient.

"This is fine. I'm fine! You can just stop right here." It's Candace, come back from the dye study of her Hickman catheter. She wants to get off her carrier in the hallway rather than immediately outside her room. The escort is older than I am, with thick glasses and gray hair. He argues with her in a monotone.

"This is policy. I take you back to your room. No getting off in the corridor."

"Stop. Stop!" Candace glides off the right side of the stretcher, making a little hop to get both feet solidly on the ground. "There's my room." She points to it. "I'm close enough and I'm getting off."

The escort looks up at the door to her room. "That's your room?"

"That's my room." He frowns, makes a *tshcck* noise with his mouth.

"OK. Here's the chart." He hands it to me. "You're back at your room." He looks at Candace, then he turns the carrier around and slowly pushes it up the hallway.

"They weren't at all nice down there. Not at all, but at least now I know my line is working."

"That's good. I'm glad." I try to smile but feel sure I look insincere.

"My cousin had to take her son to pick up his car from the shop but she'll be back soon. I'm going to give the room one more going over *now*." I don't argue. I can call Candace paranoid and a germ-o-phobe, but she's not necessarily wrong to want to sanitize her room. The truth probably is that I just wish she weren't so public about it

Another fifteen minutes, another set of vitals. This time Mr. Hampton is sitting upright in bed instead of curled up on top of it. He's also got color in his cheeks and it's not a flush, like a medication reaction, but a gentle pink that looks like health. I ask Trace if he and Stephen propped up Mr. Hampton themselves.

"No, he just sat up a few minutes ago by himself."

Hmmmm. I'm not sure what to make of that. His oxygen saturation is also staying at 100 percent without any fluctuations, which suggests he may not need supplemental oxygen and can breathe room air and be fine. "Let's take off the oxygen and see how he does." Mr. Hampton himself nods in agreement. I turn the oxygen flow down to zero, then take the plastic prongs of the nasal cannula out of Mr. Hampton's nostrils and remove the rest of the cannula from behind his ears. His eyes focus on what I'm doing with my hands, following along as I hang the now-discarded tubing off the oxygen flow meter on the wall.

Stephen is telling a story about a trip the three of them took and Mr. Hampton listens attentively.

I re-check his oxygen saturation level to see how he's doing on room air. The pulse-ox machines are addicting because of their speed: good news and bad are quickly revealed with a two-digit number. Now off supplemental oxygen, Mr. Hampton fluctuates between 97 and 99 percent. Wow. That would be normal for anyone. I look back on the computer to check his previous oxygen levels, but he was only here for half a day yesterday and got put on O_2 right away so they're not helpful.

"Was he on oxygen at home?" I ask Trace.

"Oh no. Never."

I pucker my eyebrows. "Do you know why they started the oxygen here?"

"He was short of breath." Trace tells me. "Just felt like he couldn't get enough air." Now he takes over the story of their vacation, talking about having to portage a canoe: emptying it out and then carrying it and its contents overland. He gestures with both hands and makes sure to include me by catching my eye as he talks.

"That was hard work," Mr. Hampton says, chuckling. I'm so surprised I flinch. He understands. He speaks! He laughs!

Trace and Stephen laugh along with him and I realize that Mr. Hampton's not a frail old man at the beginning of a tragic decline. He's a lively septuagenarian whose manner for the past few days has been anomalous.

I can't explain to myself what's happening. Rituxan cannot work this fast, or if it does, it tends to cause serious problems. Could it have been the drugs he got beforehand? His Tylenol, Benadryl, and an intravenous steroid? Maybe, but I've given that drug combination to lots of people without it miraculously restoring their health.

I take his vital signs again and his numbers are perfect. He holds out his arm for the blood pressure cuff, smiles as I slide the thermometer under his tongue. I don't understand it, and I can't explain it, but it's good.

"I'll be back," I tell them. Trace mouths, "Thank you."

Stephen bends forward in his chair, ". . . I only have to outrun the bear," he says, and Trace laughs at the old joke. Mr. Hampton leans back on the bed, his breath coming without effort. I quietly close the door on my way out.

I myself don't believe in miracles, but being pleasantly surprised, in the hospital or out, is always welcome. It feels good to think that the love of family or friends can bring on a turnaround that science can't explain. Liz Tilberis, the editor-in-chief of *Harper's Bazaar*, had ovarian cancer and in her memoir *No Time to Die*, she tells us that a phone call from Princess Diana raised her platelet count, making it possible for her to leave the hospital and spend the weekend in the Hamptons near the beach. "I believe the princess was single-handedly responsible for getting me home, and no one will ever convince me otherwise," she writes. Princess Diana called and Liz Tilberis's platelet count went up. Mr. Hampton needed oxygen and was confused until his son visited and they traded memories and jokes about past travels. My rational mind doesn't believe getting better can be that easy, but hospitals are full of stories just like Tilberis's, and whether it's coincidence or the power of connection, the positive effects are real.

In the hallway Doris, the minister, is waiting for me at my medcart. "We said a prayer in case she doesn't make it."

I frown. It sounds so sad.

"No, it was nice," she says, like someone at a different kind of job might say, "I just finished the meeting with Thompson. It went well." That's why I like her; she's both spiritual and down-to-earth. Doris seems to adapt her faith to the occasion while keeping her belief just as strong. I find that flexibility comforting.

"It's lucky they have a nurse who's concerned about their spiritual welfare as well as their physical," she tells me before she leaves.

I never thought about it that way before and it's a nice compliment. However, truth is, they wanted a minister, so I got a minister; any other nurse would have done the same. It's what we do. I once bought a newspaper for a patient because she was bored and wanted one. On a different shift, in the evening, I almost cried with frustration because I couldn't get jam for a dying patient nibbling on dry toast. Another nurse on the floor regularly brought in Fruity Pebbles cereal for a patient who wouldn't eat anything else.

"I gotta go," Doris says, heading up the hall to minister to someone else. I watch her springy walk and wonder if I should have asked her to say a prayer for me before she left.

As I watch her leave I see one of our phlebotomists come down the hall. "I'm here to draw blood for Fields," she says, pulling her metal cart filled with tubes, tourniquets, needles, and labels to a stop.

"What do you have?"

She hands me three labels for three tubes of blood to match Sheila's blood type with our existing stocks of red blood cells in case she needs a transfusion. Two of those tubes are supposed to be drawn now and the third one thirty minutes later. If the tubes and the blood types match there's no question it's the same blood from the same person.

I'm guessing that someone (phlebotomist? nurse?) at some time made a mistake: The wrong patient's name was put on a tube of blood that was sent to be typed and screened. As a result of this mistake, a patient's blood was "typed"—labeled A+ or O- —incorrectly, which is a serious error because transfusing someone with the wrong type blood could make her very sick.

The problem is, although drawing and sending an extra "third tube" of blood may be an excellent safeguard against errors in blood typing it's completely impractical. The phlebotomists cover the entire hospital and don't have time to take blood from a specific patient and then return in half an hour to repeat the process. So, all three tubes of blood get drawn at the same time and one gets held back and sent down later. That tube of blood becomes the "third tube" even though it was drawn at the same time as all the others and thus in no way ensures the safety of blood typing in the hospital.

True to form, the phlebotomist looks at me guiltily and explains, "Um, I'm just gonna draw all three of these type and screens now. No way I can be back here in thirty minutes."

I look at the metal clipboard on her cart and see that the lined top sheet of paper is entirely filled with patient names and the blood work they need.

"Just send that third tube a few minutes later. It's what we always do."

I nod. This is how the new rule plays and it's a classic hospital work-around. Besides, we already have procedures in place to ensure 100 percent accuracy in labeling of blood tubes and if everyone followed those rules, mistakes wouldn't be an issue. A type and screen requires that two staff members check the patient's name and ID number against the preprinted labels from the lab. We're also supposed to physically attach those verified labels to the filled tubes of blood in the patient's room. These two steps make mislabeling a tube of blood impossible. Adding in a new rule is unlikely to encourage stringency in staff members who are either careless or too busy to carry out the required checks, but layering on protocols is a standard way hospitals respond to mistakes.

The phlebotomist goes into Sheila's room to draw her blood and I follow her. She turns on the light and Sheila, her sister, and brother-in-law all blink at the sudden illumination.

"I'm here to draw your blood," she says, all business. "Let's see what you've got." She bends down to Sheila's right arm, then runs her fingers expertly up and down it. "Here's a good one." She snatches a tourniquet off her cart and ties it tightly around Sheila's upper arm. I see a vein to the right of her elbow crease pop out.

I pick up Sheila's left wrist so that I can read off her ID bracelet. "Sorry about this," I say quietly. "How's your pain?" She shakes her head and closes her eyes.

"Go ahead," the phlebotomist says. She's holding up the label for Sheila's type and screen and peers at it closely while I read Sheila's name and medical record number off the ID band on her wrist.

"Yeah. They match." She quickly writes her initials and the

time and date on the labels, then hands them to me to do the same.

"We need to check her blood type before the surgery," I explain as the phlebotomist lines up her tubes for blood and unwraps a needle. Sheila's sister nods, accepting.

"I'm gonna let you work," I tell the phlebotomist, giving a wan smile as she slides the needle into Sheila's vein. Sheila shuts her eyes shut tight, then lets out a loud breath.

"Hold on, Ms. Fields, I need three tubes," the phlebotomist says as I leave.

In the hallway I check the time on my computer screen: 6:10 p.m. Ninety more minutes to two hours or less in the shift, depending on how late I have to stay tying up loose ends. I can do this. There's a fair amount of research suggesting that twelve-hour shifts for nurses are dangerous for patients and lead to burnout for nurses. I like the continuity of twelves—knowing I have someone for a whole day—but these days are very long and I don't know if I can sustain this pace year after year. I also wonder if my patients benefit from having the same nurse over twelve hours—what we call "continuity of care"—or if they would be better off with a nurse who's fresh every eight hours.

The metal dietary cart comes into my pod and I catch an aroma of food. It's bland enough that I don't end up feeling hungry myself. As the meal delivery woman slides out the dinner trays and delivers them to Mr. Hampton and Candace I click on my computer tabs, looking for new orders. Thirty separate items pop up for Candace. The oncology fellow, Yong Sun, must have put them in; everything she needs before the transplant. I close my eyes.

The phone rings and I let it go. Once. Twice. Three times. A fourth ring. "T., what are you so busy doing that you're not answering your phone?"

It's the secretary and for the second time that day her friendly pestering irritates me. At this moment I find her irrepressible cheerfulness annoying.

"T., tell the truth. Were you in the bathroom?"

"Yep. I dropped the phone in and it took me a minute to fish it out."

She snorts into the phone. "Is the room ready for Irving? I'm supposed to call and check."

I glance through the door to Dorothy's old room. "It looks ready."

"*Looks* ready? T., after Candace Moore and her crazy shower curtain you need to get in there and make *sure* it's clean."

So now we're doing housekeeping's job. I step into the room, wipe my finger across the aluminum brackets on the wall that hold oxygen and suction. No dust comes off. I look under the bed and the floor is shiny—no bacteria balls. "It's clean."

"Great."

What I wouldn't give for a moment where nothing in my world rings, dings, or alarms.

Then Sheila's call light turns on and I check my record of when she last got pain medicine. She's overdue. I wonder if she was hurting when I was in the room with the phlebotomist and didn't tell me. She's also worried she's going to die, if not tonight, then soon, and she's being stuck with a needle.

And like that I'm back. I turn myself around, go to her room, open her door and reach in to turn off the call light. "Do you need more Dilaudid?" I ask her, my voice steady and clear.

This is what I'm here for.

CHAPTER 11

Revolving Door

After going through the usual procedure—pass code, accu-dose code, count, and confirm—I've got the Dilaudid. I check the concentration on the vial one more time, draw up the drug, and dilute it in 10 ml of saline. Check the volume. Drop the glass vial into the sharps' container attached to my medcart. In nursing school they told us that addicts have been known to dig empty vials out of the trash to get whatever drops of narcotic are left inside clinging to the walls of the empty syringes. I have no idea if that's true but I treat empty narcotic vials as if they're contraband.

I go into Sheila's room. The phlebotomist is finishing up and surreptitiously hands me the "third tube" for Sheila's type and screen. "I'll send these to the lab right now," she says overly loudly, holding up the other tubes.

Sheila's sister looks up briefly when I come in, then returns her gaze to the floor. Sheila's eyes are closed, her lips held tight together from the pain. I pick up her left arm and shoot the Dilaudid into her IV, follow it up with a saline flush.

"Did the pain get away from you?" I ask.

"It was OK," she says, closing her eyes tightly, "and then it"—she gasps—"wasn't."

She looks up at me now, apologetically. "I need to pee."

"Of course. Can you roll toward me on this side? It's less walking then." She nods, then slowly rolls to her left. Her eyes flitter open, then close again. She pants.

I didn't ask her to rate her pain with ten being "the worst pain ever." Some people, and Sheila is probably one of them, could have an arm half cut off and would cry out "six," covered in sweat, straining to make their voices sound normal. Patients like that also rarely ask for pain medicine before they're in agony because they believe their pain never rises to the level of deserving to be treated. Although I explained the physiological reasons for staying ahead of her pain to Sheila, I should have realized she might not follow my suggestion. The trick with a patient such as her is to watch her face, see how she moves, or doesn't. Faces rarely lie about pain, but sometimes you have to look closely and today I haven't done that. I was persuaded by Sheila's stoicism, fooled into thinking she needed less pain medication than she probably did. Trouble is, the joke's not on me—she's the one who has suffered.

Pain is awful. It hurts. But narcotics, the drugs that best treat pain, come with their own patina of shame, even here in the hospital. There are health care workers who reserve a special kind of scorn for drug abusers, probably because we've all heard stories about being burned by an addict: a patient someone went the extra mile for only to discover the patient wasn't actually in pain, she just wanted to get high. Patients with chronic pain are often labeled "drug-seeking." Sickle-cell patients, who live lives filled with pain and during disease crises can get relief only from large doses of opioids, sometimes get dismissed as junkies. Do we in health care hate the need for narcotics due to their high potential for abuse or is it the pain itself we find outrageous? We can't see it, can't test for it objectively. We're taught "Pain is whatever the patient says it is," but then we don't believe our patients, and in that lack of belief we miss the message of pain. People born without a sense of pain—a rare affliction called congenital insensitivity to pain—are in constant danger. Pain is a neural explosion telling us that something is very wrong. Today I missed the full import of Sheila's pain.

"Do you think you can stand up to go to the bathroom? Let me help you." I reach down for Sheila's arm when my phone rings.

"This is the OR. We're ready for your patient Fields."

"Oh." I look at my watch. "You're early." I don't intend to sound accusing but I do.

"We had a cancellation. And they wanted to get this one down ASAP."

This is good news for Sheila, but my work for her isn't done yet. She needs to pee and there's paperwork to finish.

"That's the OR," I tell her and her family, hanging up my phone. "They're ready for her."

"Ready? But it's early," her sister says.

"They were able to make room for her. So I just need to complete her paperwork, after she goes to the bathroom, that is." I smile at Sheila, whose eyes are slits.

"No. We'll get her to the bathroom," her sister says. "You go and get her ready." She stands up and her husband stands up, too.

"Are you sure? Can you manage?"

"We'll be fine. We're fine. She has to get down to that operating room."

I nod. "Call if you need me." Back at my medcart I pull up Sheila's pre-op form. More boxes to check and click.

What are her vital signs? Does she have allergies? Was there a history and physical done within three days and is it on the chart? Have her belongings been safely stowed? That last question doesn't seem so important. Sheila could die on the table. Does it matter where her clothes end up? But of course it does. Even in the midst of calamity ordinary details must be attended to. It reminds us that life goes on.

One of the odder experiences I had in the hospital also revolved around a patient's property, though property of a more personal nature. I walked into a patient's room at 8 a.m., start of shift, having never met her or any member of her family before. A tall thin woman with a very short haircut held out a denture cup to me, with the plastic lid on, and said, "These are not her teeth!"

I try to always be patient in the hospital but sometimes I get my hackles up when people are rude, and this was one of those times. I arched my eyebrows. "These are not her teeth!" the woman said again, thrusting the denture cup toward me.

"Excuse me?"

"She went down to a CT scan, returned to this room, and these are not her teeth!"

She'd said it three times now. "And you are?"

"Her daughter."

The woman standing next to her, heavier and shorter, spoke up. "I'm her daughter, too, and these are definitely not her teeth!" Just then the rounding medical team came in, all six of them. I hadn't gotten much information in report, but as the medical team started talking it became clear that the patient, a woman in her eighties, did not have long to live. She was also barely conscious.

So I put the dentures out of my mind. The patient would not be needing them. And then I got busy, just like any normal day, except a little busier than usual: phone ringing constantly, a string of time-consuming miscommunications, hands in need of holding, medications to be given, and, if I'm totally honest, lives with more promise to be tended.

At some later point in the day the daughter found me to relay a precise description of how the dentures in the cup differed from her mother's. The canines were too long, the incisors too short, or maybe it was the other way around. I took a minute, called CT, asked if they had any misplaced dentures forgotten on a counter. They reacted as if I was insane. Plus, the scan had been done the day before, when the staff at CT had been completely different. No one there now had seen the patient the day before. Learning this and thinking about it made me wonder why the night-shift nurse had not been asked about the mixed-up dentures. Maybe by the time the patient returned to the floor following the test, the family had already left for the night.

Finally at the end of the shift I had time to talk to that day's charge nurse, who made a point of being involved. She talked to the nurse-in-charge, who oversees the whole hospital. Her explanation didn't help with locating the teeth, but it was reasonable. "I don't understand," she said. "Does CT just have sets of teeth lined up waiting to be returned to patients and sometimes there's a mix-up?" The imaging center had no idea how a patient could come down for a scan and return to the floor with the wrong teeth. Why would a patient even need to have her dentures removed for a CT scan? And most important of all, why was a patient so near death having a CT scan anyway?

I punted. I gave up. I left. My shift was over, but thinking back on it now I feel ashamed of myself for walking out without having solved the problem. There was, however, nothing I could tell those daughters about their mother's teeth. I wonder if our carelessness with the dentures made the daughters think we had generally been careless with their mother, including the grim prognosis she received. Dentures are irrelevant to a hospital staff when a patient's very survival is unlikely, but relatives may look at such scenes through the other end of the telescope: If we can't keep track of someone's dentures how can we be trusted to care for her whole body?

The dentures could also have been a proxy for the mother's

life. It's a not uncommon reaction to getting very bad news about someone you love. All the pain and anger of grief focuses, like light concentrated through a magnifying glass, on some small item that absolutely does not matter. "These are not her teeth!" Two daughters' lives condensed into the contents of one cheap plastic denture cup. A mother's death is a deep, some would say irreparable, loss.

I attentively fill out the form for Sheila. No, she does not have dentures. Yes she has glasses and will leave them with her sister. No, she has nothing of value that needs to be locked up. Yes, her sister will take care of her clothes.

Our patients become like refugees, hustled from floor to floor, bed to bed, with the minimum of belongings. I finish the form and save it, look at my watch: Vital signs! I forgot. Into Mr. Hampton's room, the blood pressure cuff, the thermometer, the pulse-ox monitor. He's normal, fully and completely normal, and he, Trace, and Stephen continue to talk excitedly, this time about fly-fishing. To me there is nothing more boring than fishing, but they have so much enthusiasm it feels like fun. Their energy draws me in the same way it seems to have pumped up Mr. Hampton.

I check the time against the computer and realize I'm ten minutes late with these vitals. I go through the usual debate with myself about writing down the correct time or the actual time and then write down the actual time.

"He's good," I say, after eyeing the IV pump and tubing. The three of them stop talking long enough to absorb what I say and then return to their stories. They are self-sufficient in a way that comforts me as well as them. When a patient does so much better than expected I enjoy not being needed.

Candace's door is open and she calls out as soon as I step into the hall. "There you are! I have some questions."

Oh my goodness. Well, there's no avoiding her, so I go in, shutting the door behind me.

"So who was that doctor who came in here earlier? Yong—somebody."

She's referring to Yong Sun, the oncology fellow. I explain that he's an oncologist in training and that he'll work with the oncology attending in the hospital to manage her transplant.

"So even though I'm finally getting my transplant my regular doctor won't be here?"

"No-oo," I tell her, reluctantly. Even though our outpatient cancer center is literally across the street from the hospital, whichever physician the patient has been seeing there—sometimes for months or years—will not necessarily be involved in that patient's care once she is admitted to the hospital. The inpatient attending is supposed to check in with the patient's regular oncologist, but if that MD is not scheduled to round on that patient in the hospital then it is rare for that doc to see the patient during her stay.

This tends to be how care is managed in teaching hospitals and the idea is to use physician time efficiently, but patients dislike it for obvious reasons. They want to be seen and supervised by the MD who knows their case better than anyone else. In *How Doctors Think* Jerome Groopman writes that the individual doctor makes all the difference in how an oncology patient fares. That may or may not be true, but if it is, then why are teaching hospitals structured in this way: separating patients from their usual doctors when patients are most vulnerable? If having patients managed by a specific doctor matters, then why are secondhand reports from residents, fellows, or other attendings, considered good enough when the patient is arguably the sickest she will be?

Candace knows the usual arrangements for rounding; she's venting by pretending to be uninformed. I don't mind, though. It's very hard when patients see "their" doctor on rounds in the hallways and that MD fails to stop at their room or even say hello. I also don't have what I consider a good enough explanation for why we do things this way. The system's teaching efficiency doesn't matter to the people who are sick; all they want is for the person they know and trust to be taking care of them.

"That guy barely knew my history. I won't have a physician who doesn't know my plan for transplant taking care of me."

"And you shouldn't have to, Candace." Yong Sun is here to learn, but for Candace, getting a stem cell transplant is scary enough. We shouldn't add in worries that knowledge of patients is piecemeal. "I'll pass along the message. It may be possible to switch with an oncology fellow who's more familiar with your case. I'll try."

"Fine," she says, nodding her head definitively. "I appreciate that."

"You're welcome." In this moment I admire her. She's

willing to complain about things that so many other patients mind but don't speak up about. I add this request to my mental grocery list, written in bold and underlined.

As I step out of Candace's room the escort is holding up Sheila's chart to get my attention. It's a different one this time, the young woman who pulls her long brown hair up into a pouffy ponytail and wears a lot of eye makeup. I like her because she's friendly and patient, which is rarely true of the escorts who come from the OR. Their schedules are usually too tight for that.

"Can she walk?" She inclines her head toward Sheila's door.

"Yes, but slowly."

"Should I take the stretcher into the room?"

"No, it's OK. I'll go and get her." I'm not sure what's motivating me here. It's easier not to bring the stretcher into the room, but leaving it outside will make the transfer harder for Sheila. However, if she walks out of the room under her own steam she has set a tone of strength and determination that will, I'm hoping, endure. The operation she's being taken to will save her life and it's my belief that walking to the stretcher tonight will lead to her walking out of the hospital a few weeks later when our work is done.

There's a word for this kind of thinking: crazy. I'm not being rational. "If wishes were horses, beggars would ride," my mother often says. Well, fine. This is one wish I'm going to take out of the stable and see how far I can go on it. Once Sheila leaves here she's out of my hands. I won't be there to explain the diagnostic mistake, hold her hand and wipe her brow, or say,

Please, *please* be careful with her. I trust the people I work with in the hospital, but they're not me.

I open the door to Sheila's room. This is the moment when I have to let go. "They'll take good care of you. You're in good hands now." I must say good-bye with confidence, wish her all the best.

Her sister and brother-in-law flank her as she sits on the bed. Her breaths come deep and rough and she's squinting as if to block out the pain. The last dose of Dilaudid hasn't helped much. "We can move the stretcher in here if it hurts too much to walk." I offer.

But Sheila herself shakes her head no at the idea of the stretcher being brought to her and instead slowly rises from the bed. Eyes closed, she bends forward just slightly and then straightens up. Her sister takes one arm, her brother-in-law the other. I walk in front of them, pulling the IV pump and holding out one arm toward Sheila as if to catch her should she slip and fall.

We move slowly. It's maybe four feet from the bed to the door, four feet from the door to the stretcher. The time feels infinite. With every step Sheila lets out a contained "Hummph."

Another nurse would call for the stretcher now, insist she shouldn't walk. Not me. And maybe it's not magical thinking. Maybe I believe in the power of normalcy.

At no time was this principle clearer to me than when the Twin Towers fell in New York on September 11, 2001. We were living in Princeton, New Jersey, close enough that what happened felt very real. Our daughters were just two and a half, our son five years old. I'd been doing research in the Princeton Public Library for the microbiology class I was taking as a prerequisite for nursing school. We had to write a short paper about West Nile virus.

I was reading articles, taking notes when I noticed a cluster of people in the library's lobby all watching TV. Curious, I went over. "A plane flew into one of the towers," one of the librarians told me, her voice low and tight, nervous in a way that seemed out of proportion. I didn't understand. A small prop plane went wildly off course. Odd. Dangerous for the people involved, of course, but no more.

And then the first tower fell, on the TV screen right in front of me, all one hundred and ten stories of it collapsing into a giant pile of cement and fire and toxic dust. The second tower fell soon after. In my memory, the collapses are separated by only a few minutes, although the south tower fell at 9:58 a.m. and the north tower at 10:28 a.m., thirty minutes later. Afterwards I went back to my research and methodically finished up my notes, thinking, *Things aren't going to feel normal for a long time; I want one more dose of normal before that begins.*

But of course there's no way to be sure that Sheila herself preferred a dose of normal over having the stretcher brought to her. She's such a stoic she would never say she couldn't walk, especially since I presented walking to the stretcher as the first choice option. Hmmm. In my need to help her feel indomitable, have I inadvertently caused her pointless pain? I'll never know.

Once Sheila makes it to the stretcher it's almost too high for her to get up on and this one doesn't adjust. What genius designed these stretchers? Sheila's not tall but she's not that short, either. "I'll go grab a step," the escort says, hurrying off as Sheila stands with her back to the stretcher, pulling in long, shallow breaths and letting them out with a raggedy exhale. She's not sweating, so the walk didn't completely tax her.

The escort returns quickly—"Here you go!"—putting a one-step footstool behind Sheila's feet, then maneuvering the carrier just slightly backward to give her a little more room. The brake locks back in place with a loud *ka-thunk*. It takes the four of us to get her on. Sheila's sister has one arm, her brother-in-law the other. I'm reaching in, my head close to hers, my arms under her armpits and the escort is standing on the other side of the stretcher waiting to help. I count out loud "one-two-three," just like on TV, and we lift, except in real life it requires actual exertion, not just looking cool.

It works and we get Sheila onto the stretcher. She gives out a low moan, her eyes tightly shut.

"We're going to lay you down now," I tell her, making sure the IV tubing is out and away from her body. She doesn't need that to be pulling on her arm.

I ease her back on one side, her brother-in-law on the other, while her sister picks up her legs. We get her flat and she sighs and opens her eyes. "Better?" She shrugs.

I look at her. This is the moment when she will leave my care for good. Mine may be the last familiar hospital face she sees before she goes under and I want her to remember it as calm and present.

"I have to give you a hug," I say.

"And a kiss," she says in return, surprising me. What kind of a kiss, I wonder, is this?

Kisses in the hospital, real kisses, are as the six pomegranate seeds must have been to Persephone in the underworld: rare, enticing, a taste of life impossible to resist when you're stuck in hell.

A few years ago the wife of a patient who had just died stood in the hallway and kissed me on the lips over and over again. "You're an angel," she murmured.

Well, no, but I had made sure he could die in the hospital on our floor, which had been his home and hers for the last few months. Reimbursement rules said he should go to hospice, which would involve a bumpy ride in an ambulance to deliver him and his wife to an unfamiliar place with nurses and doctors they didn't know. He'd had tubes inserted so that his urine drained into bags outside his body and they never worked right. The end of his life was pain.

I made my case for not moving him with the nurse practitioner in palliative care. I don't remember what I said. There was no medical reason for keeping him in the hospital—the guy was dying and people can and do die anywhere. The argument for moving him came down to money. Hospitals get reimbursed at a lower rate for hospice patients than those who are expected to live. He'd be using a bed the hospital could get more cash for.

I, however, didn't give a damn about that. Either I persuaded the nurse practitioner of the wisdom of his staying or she was colluding with me, but we got the patient switched over to hospice in the hospital. It was our biggest room, too, supposedly for VIPs, with extra space for a sitting area, sort of like a suite room in a hotel, with a couch. The hospital bed was hidden behind enclosing curtains. What that wife had done for her husband over months as he fought the inevitable—she deserved at least a sofa and maybe a medal, too, for extreme selflessness without complaint. I know. I was there. She was the real angel.

I look at Sheila, put my arms around her neck as she lies on the stretcher, and go to kiss her on the cheek, but she moves and we kiss on the lips. Sealed with a kiss. Kiss and tell. A Judas kiss. The kiss of life.

The escort takes hold of the carrier and pushes her up the hall with her sister and brother in law following behind carrying her few belongings even though we could have transported them later. Away and away with nothing of her left in the room. *Good luck*, I think to myself, but I don't say it out loud. Instead I swallow, and my phone rings.

"T., your admission is here."

"Who?"

"Your admission. Irving. You've been waiting half the day for him! Wake up," she laughs over the phone.

"Oh. Right." My mind feels like a battleship trying to turn in shallow water. Irving. "Send him back once he's checked in."

And then I remember the final thing I need to do for Sheila. I call Akash, Peter's surgical resident, my neighbor. "She's on her way," I tell him, just as he had asked me to do.

I don't ask if they'll take her tonight or if she's just going down to be prepped by anesthesia. I had put in my pitch to

Peter already and now all I can do is hope the surgery happens as soon as it's safe for Sheila and not any later. Besides, it's not Akash's decision and he may not know right now anyway. Even Peter may not know, since doing the surgery depends on Sheila's clotting time, which is tricky to evaluate because of her disease and the Argatroban.

I check the last box on her pre-op form—the one that records when she left the floor—and stick my hand in my pocket, feeling the "third tube" of Sheila's blood that the phlebotomist gave me for her type and screen. Right. I had forgotten. I walk up to our pneumatic tube station and send the tube to the lab, more or less thirty minutes after the other two tubes went.

I'm back at my medcart when two burly EMTs push a loaded stretcher through the double doors that separate my part of the floor from the front section. Then I hear Irving's whispery voice: "OK now. We're here at the hospital now. OK."

"Hi, Irving. It's Theresa, but you may not remember me."

He's strapped down, but he looks up toward me. "I might remember," he says, as the EMT hands me an envelope filled with paperwork and they wheel him into Dorothy's old room.

CHAPTER 12

End of Shift

You guys OK in here?" The EMTs are lower-
ing Irving's stretcher, unstrapping him, putting the side rails
down.

"Oh yeah, we know Irving." EMTs have a reputation for
being adrenaline junkies, hardened to the job, and they see a lot:
people dead from sudden heart attacks, gunshot victims with
clothing covered in blood, accidental overdoses by the young.
The adrenaline rush is good, I imagine, and the ability to stay
calm when all external signals are screaming "panic!" must be
gratifying, too. The pulseless body, the crying wife, could become intoxicating; called in daily to traverse the border between
life and death. Licensed to save. But that kind of grind could
wear on a person because there would be many times when the
patient couldn't be rescued.

It's probably a relief to ferry around someone like Irving, and they seem to really know him. They may have taken him to his outpatient chemo appointments and his doctor visits, becoming part of the family he doesn't have. EMTs' talk can be rough, their manner brusque, but it seems obvious they care about the people they're responsible for. After all, why else would they do the job?

My daughter Sophia, when she was seven, swallowed a nickel. She'd put it in her mouth the way kids do, maybe to explore the impressions on its smooth surfaces, trace the roundness of its edges with her tongue. It was in her mouth and then down her throat when she called out. I had just started nursing school, but knew that if she could talk she could breathe. Her airway wasn't blocked. I also knew to call 911 and soon enough the ambulance came, bringing two EMTs. One, a woman, strikingly pretty with dark skin and hair in small tight braids, fit the tough EMT stereotype. But the other one, a guy, youngish with sandy blond hair, had a gentleness that surprised me.

They told us our daughter was fine, but after talking into the walkie-talkies strapped to their chests the guy, oh so softly, said, "We're gonna have to take a ride." Crap. It was nine o'clock at night. I was hoping to avoid the hospital. But, again, I'd been in nursing school long enough that I didn't argue. If they wanted to take us in, I figured there was a reason.

My daughter and I, she in her footie pajamas because she'd been getting ready for bed, went downstairs to get into the ambulance. Rudyard Kipling's story "Rikki-Tikki-Tavi" was sitting out and I grabbed it. It was a good pick. Rikki-Tikki is a brave little mongoose. To protect his adopted British colonial family in India he must kill two full size cobras, who are husband and wife, and destroy all their eggs before the new little cobras hatch. He gets some help from other animals, but Rikki-Tikki is the hero of the story, constantly cautioning himself to stay on guard and figure out the best way to win a fight.

The kindly EMT sat in the back of the ambulance with my daughter and me and listened while I read: "This is the story of the great war that Rikki-Tikki-Tavi fought, all by himself . . . ." When we arrived at the hospital it felt too soon; I was only two-thirds of the way through the book. "I'd like to hear what ends up happening to Rikki-Tikki-Tavi," the EMT said before he lifted my daughter, wrapped in a thin but enormous white blanket, out of the ambulance and deposited her, like a princess on a chair in the waiting room of the emergency department at Pittsburgh Children's Hospital.

"It is impossible for a mongoose to stay frightened for very long," I had read, and the EMT seemed to like that idea. Long, long after my daughter got the X-ray showing the nickel wasn't lodged in her esophagus and the whole event became just another family story, I thought about finding that EMT and giving him his very own copy of "Rikki-Tikki-Tavi," but I'd never even learned his name.

"Here, I'll help you," I tell the EMTs today. "We always like having Irving on the floor."

Unstrapped, Irving gets himself up off the stretcher and walks over to the chair in the room. It's not one of the good armchairs, but he sits down in it with an expression of placid contentment. "That's nice." His voice is a whisper we can barely hear as he rubs his hands back and forth a few times over the armrests, satisfied in a way that suggests life has lost its ability to disappoint.

"OK, Irving," one of the EMTs calls out, his voice overly loud but friendly. "We'll be back to get you when you're ready to come home." They pull the stretcher up to waist height, making it easier to push, and head out.

"Is this Irving Mooney?" a young woman in a long white coat looks cautiously through the door. She must be the intern assigned to Irving. She's petite and her straight black hair ends in a modern stacked cut just at the nape of her neck. She comes into the room, extends her hand to Irving. "I'm Meredith."

Irving doesn't seem to see her hand, or else doesn't understand why she's holding it out to him, but he nods slowly, looking up.

"And you have a rectal abscess, right?"

"A . . . what?" He cocks his head to one side.

"A rectal abscess. A sore, um, on your bum."

"Oh, yes. On my backside." He turns a little, angling his right side out toward Meredith and me. Then he reaches back with his right hand and points to a spot on his lower back just above his waist. "It hurts . . . off and on."

Meredith frowns. "I'm confused. Your back or your backside? Your back or your rear end?" She says each word distinctly.

"My backside. Here—" He angles the left side of his body away from us and points to his right side again, explaining in that low soft voice, "Here—it's on my back. Right here." Then he straightens and sits normally in the chair, his hands folded one over the other in his lap.

Another time when Irving was admitted to the hospital his scrotum was badly swollen, which is unusual but happens more than the average man might like to think. It's embarrassing and, I've heard, pretty uncomfortable. During morning rounds that day Irving told the medical team, "I've got this problem with my balls," in a voice so soothing it surprised me to realize what he'd actually said.

"Meredith!" Another woman, a little older, taller, also wearing a long white coat, comes into Irving's room. "Is this the rectal abscess?"

"Um, no. He says it's on his back."

"His back?"

"The side of his back." She walks over to Irving and points to the right side of his back.

"So, not a rectal abscess at all?"

Meredith shakes her head no. It's one of those moments when the hospital is like that childhood game, Telephone. I always wondered if some kid passing on the whispered message deliberately changed it to make sure the game worked and was funny, but I've seen it happen often enough in the hospital: the side of the back becomes the backside, which becomes the rear end, which somehow becomes the rectum. Good thing we don't need a scan to find out the truth for Irving; all we have to do is look.

"Mr. Mooney, I'm Eileen, the resident on this case. I'm working with Meredith and we need to see the abscess—the sore—on your back. Is that OK with you?" She's friendlier than when she first came into the room and I wonder if she's relieved to be dealing with an infected lesion in a much less intimate location.

"Fine, fine." Irving seems to be confirming something for himself more than talking to Eileen, but she doesn't slow down.

"Good! Because the sooner we see it, the sooner we'll know what we're dealing with." She turns to me. "Are you his nurse?"

I look at my watch. "Only for about forty more minutes."

"You can go. We've got this." I look at her. *You can go.* Am I being dismissed or given a breather? She doesn't seem rude, just purposeful, not unlike my behavior toward the EMTs who dropped Irving off.

I nod at the two of them. "Call me if you need anything—if he needs anything."

"Sure," Eileen says. Turning back to Irving: "Now if you can lie on the bed, Mr. Mooney."

Chuckling to myself about the "rectal abscess" mix-up, I close the door on my way out. Candace's call light is on in the hallway, but so is Mr. Hampton's. I step into his room first.

"Everything OK in here?"

Trace's head is thrown back in a laugh and I see that even his teeth are perfect. "The call light's on. Did you need me?" I step into the room and shut the door. That way I don't hear the ring accompanying Candace's call light and I won't see it. Out of sight, out of mind. If she were really in trouble her cousin would probably have burst out of the room yelling for help, or that's what I tell myself.

Trace collects himself, looks up at the light flashing on the wall. "Oh, no, we're fine. It must have been an accident."

I walk over to the bed and fish out the remote from under Mr. Hampton's knee.

Mr. Hampton shakes his head. "Mistake," he says.

"Hey—sorry," Trace tells me.

"No problem. Like I said, I'd rather come in and have it be nothing than walk into an emergency because you didn't call." I reach behind the bed to turn off the alarm. "I'll be leaving soon; it's the end of shift. Can I get anyone anything before I go?"

"Oh. No. Nothing," Trace says. "But thanks for everything." He gives me a sincere look, without the movie-star smile.

I'm ready to brush off his gratitude, to say I'm only doing my job, when I bite my tongue. "You are very welcome," I say, taking all three of them in with a glance.

Candace's call light is off once I get back in the hallway. The aide must have answered it. *That's a relief,* I think, and then I remember the chair. Sheila's comfy armchair, the one her brother-in-law spent all day sitting in; I was going to give it to Candace as a kind of peace offering and because it would be a nice thing to do.

I think over what else I have to get done. I recorded report on Mr. Hampton once it was clear he would do OK with the Rituxan. Candace doesn't have much going on and Irving just got here, so report for him will be easy. No need to do voice care on Sheila, because even if they don't operate tonight she'll almost definitely go to ICU instead of returning here, and Dorothy is long gone. I'll give face-to-face reports—what we call "verbals"—for Candace and Irving. We're supposed to al-ways record change of shift information for the oncoming nurse, but with new admissions we often don't. It's easier just to talk to the nurse taking over.

It's 6:55 p.m. I need to be in the conference room in five minutes. Moving fast, I grab some Clorox wipes out of the dis-penser on the wall and go into Sheila's room to wipe down the chair. Candace will wipe it down again of course but I don't want to offend her by introducing a dirty chair into her clean room.

The chairs are big and look solid but they're actually very light. Disinfection accomplished, I push the chair out of Sheila's room to Candace's door. I knock.

Two voices call out, "Come in."

Opening the door I see Candace and her cousin eating pizza. When did that pizza get here? It must have been when I was in Irving's room. I catch a whiff of the pepperoni and cheese and I feel a twinge in my stomach. No surprise.

"Hey. I thought you might like one of our primo armchairs." I gesture toward it. "I just cleaned it. Another patient had it but she's gone to the OR and won't be coming back."

Candace stands up to look at the big brown chair. I can't tell what she's thinking. "I've got a chair in the room right now."

"I know, but this one's a lot more comfortable and I can trade yours. We move furniture around all the time."

"Can it be cleaned with bleach?"

"Uh-huh. Just like all the others."

She stands there for a minute longer, saying nothing. "OK.

That's great. But we can do it." Following some unspoken command, Candace's cousin hops up and starts moving the smaller armchair out of Candace's room while Candace takes the comfy chair and maneuvers it inside the door. "We'll have to wipe it down," she says aggressively. Then she stops pushing and looks at me. "Thank you."

"You bet," I tell her, taking the old chair from her cousin so that I can put it in Sheila's room.

In the conference room the nurse taking over for me has her papers and is sitting down to listen to voice care. I tell her she'll be getting verbals for my two admissions and she nods, punching in the right codes to hear report on Mr. Hampton.

Maya the aide, who's heading into a double shift, is eating a piece of pizza. Each pepperoni has an opalescent drop of grease inside it, but looking at it makes my mouth water.

"Where'd you get that?" I try to sound nonchalant.

"Candace," she says while chewing, and for a minute I feel bad they didn't offer me a slice when I went in.

"She said she would have given you some, but you must not have heard the call light."

"Oh." I feel my face fall. I'm suddenly that hungry.

"So I asked for a piece for you anyway." She holds up another plate, covered with an unfolded napkin, and underneath the napkin is a second piece of pepperoni pizza, also shiny with grease. I don't even really like pepperoni, but the happiness I feel about this cold oily piece of pizza blooms like a tea flower dropped in hot water.

"You are wonderful." I take the plate from her, lean up

against the computer table in the conference room and start eating. The pizza hits me like a drug as I chew and swallow, barely pausing.

"Did she need anything?"

"Nah!" Maya says. She takes an index finger and circles it around in the air next to her temple—the universal symbol for crazy. "She's batshit."

I laugh. I ought to tell her she's wrong, that Candace has been through a lot, that any of us might react to being hospitalized the way she has. But I don't. I just eat.

The nurse taking over for me finishes report on Mr. Hampton and clicks off her phone. "So he's getting Rituxan until two in the morning?" she snaps. The thought of taking several sets of vital signs during the night must be annoying.

I raise my hands, palms up, a placating gesture. "He's doing fine with it."

She sighs. "Rituxan, Candace Moore, an admission who just got here, Beth's patient up front who can't walk and needs to pee constantly and whatever other train wreck comes our way tonight since I'll get the next admission, too."

"Candace is content right now and nothing starts for her until tomorrow. She came early because she was worried about her central line—which is fine—so no worries there. Irving should need only IV antibiotics and fluids." More placating. "And I'm here tomorrow," I tell her, which makes giving report in the morning easier since we usually get our previous patients back.

"I just don't want to be here," she says, "It's my fifth twelve this week."

"Your fifth nightshift this week!"

"Well, we're short because they haven't approved a new hire for nights and the truth is, I can use the money. Our furnace is on its last legs."

Now I get it. She's exhausted and broke.

I give quick verbal reports on Candace and Irving and she takes notes. The storm of her frustration has passed and she doesn't even jump on me when she sees the list of new orders for Irving, which are more or less the standard package for his particular problem: insert an IV, administer evening medications, treat his abscess with two different intravenous antibiotics, but also consult infectious disease to make sure we're not missing anything, take vital signs every four hours, record his fluid intake and output, infuse normal saline at 150 ml/hour, and serve him a "regular" diet. Since Irving is stable, there's no urgency.

Beth walks by the conference room and gives a small wave. "Almost done," she says, smiling.

"Hey, I'm gonna go see Ray," I tell my replacement. "I'll be in his room if you need me." She's in work mode now and waves the suggestion away. "I'll be fine," she tells me.

Ray's alone in his room, reading *No Country for Old Men* by Cormac McCarthy and I ask him if it's a good book. I've never read anything by Cormac McCarthy despite how much I like the repeating hard "c's" in his cowboy-Irish name.

Ray says the book is good, then asks me if I saw the movie version, which won Best Picture in 2008.

"No. The previews made me think it would upset me." That sounds so lame. I'm an oncology nurse; I should be tougher. But to me the movie looked nihilistic—lots of violence with no point or moral behind it. I can read about such things, but seeing them, even in movies that I know aren't true, disturbs me. I guess I want to believe that at our core humans are always moral and caring.

"The movie was good," he says, "but try the book. All his books are good." He speaks deliberately, as if he has all the time in the world, as if we're back in that coffee shop where we met only a few weeks ago. So often with patients I talk with them only about their illness because I think that's what they need. But it seems like Ray wants to talk about books and movies instead of leukemia.

"I'll buy it," I tell him. "Then I'll let you know how it is."

"Well, I'll be here," he says, leaning back into the bed, running his clasped hands over his hair.

"Hey, where's Liz? Is everything OK at her job?"

"She's out getting dinner. She hates the food here." He pauses for a second to think. "Me, too, but it's free." He looks rueful and turns his eyes away from me. Then he re-collects his calm and answers my question.

"Liz's job is cool. They needed her to come in and plan for the next few weeks. You know, patient schedules, who's covering whom."

"So she's not going to be fired for being here with you?"

"Nah. Nothing like that. Not even close." He looks away again and I'm not sure what to think. If there were work issues this morning I guess they've been resolved, which is good. I would hate to be confronted with a choice between my husband and my job.

Ray's work has been unbelievably generous to him and Liz. It's a tradition among firefighters, at least in Pittsburgh, to cover for members who get sick. Individual volunteers from different crews around the city signed up for each of Ray's twenty-four-hour shifts. They worked, but Ray got the money, so his leukemia diagnosis didn't also lead to a sudden loss of income or health insurance.

Ray himself admitted that reading philosophy and post-modern novels on shift made him an oddball, but looking out for each other was integral to the culture of the job. His crew, some of whom might not have related to him that much, contributed further by buying dinner for every volunteer who took one of Ray's shifts and Ray found out about the free dinners only after he was back at work. No one from his crew or another department ever said Ray owed him anything.

While the firefighters protected Ray's livelihood, his fellow punk rockers looked after his and Liz's two kids. Their son was finishing elementary school and their daughter middle school. Liz made a schedule: every day someone would be at the house to meet the kids after school, make dinner, help with homework, hustle them into bed on time, stay the night if needed, and then send the kids off to school the next morning. Night after night after night, so that if Liz had to be in the hospital with Ray she could be. An organized rotation of self-acknowledged social misfits with piercings, blue hair, tattoos, fishnet stockings and motorcycle boots kept their family life intact.

I don't ask Ray how he feels about the relapse, if he's afraid. He must be afraid. Who wouldn't be? Afraid of getting the transplant and of not getting it. Maybe talking about Cormac McCarthy is enough. Maybe, like Sheila walking to the stretcher, Ray needs a dose of normal tonight.

Leaving his room I think I'm going home when the nurse taking over for me calls out to me at the nurses' station. "Peter Coyne is on the phone," she says, looking anxious. I wonder what's wrong. Will Sheila not get operated on tonight? Perhaps her blood still takes too long to clot.

I click the phone off hold. "It's Theresa."

"Yeah, um, we don't have a blood type yet on Sheila Field. Did the tubes get sent?"

"Yes, but the hang up might be the third tube."

"The third tube?"

"It's a rule now that if we're doing a type and screen on a new patient we have to send two separate samples of blood thirty minutes apart to make sure the right patient is typed. That second sample is the 'third tube' of blood sent."

"So the second sample wasn't sent?"

"No, it was definitely sent, but not that long ago. They may not have finished with it." I'm not telling him the third tube of blood wasn't drawn when it was supposed to be. Briefly over-dramatizing, I wonder if Sheila will not have her surgery and will die of sepsis because I bent the rule about triple-checking blood samples. But we would never allow something that awful to happen because of a mistake in procedure and the time the blood was drawn doesn't affect its processing.

"This worked a lot better when we just had anesthesia do the type and cross," Peter says, talking to himself more than to me.

"Yes, well, you know, if a system's working they decide to make it more complicated."

"And the oncologist is saying that FFP would help her, so that's a couple more hours . . . and we'll do her tonight."

It takes me a minute to understand. Tonight? He will operate on Sheila tonight. He's irritated, venting about the lab, the oncology attending, and the last-minute decision to give Sheila fresh frozen plasma (FFP), but I want to shout "Yahoo!"

Instead, "That's great," I say, with almost no affect at all, but I'm smiling now, grinning really, like Trace laughing with his dad or Beth after she talked to her daughter. It would have been so hard on Sheila and her family to postpone, possibly even dangerous, although proceeding tonight will not be easy for Peter or his team in the OR.

"Thank you," I tell him. Of course he's not operating tonight to satisfy me, but he is doing it. I feel my hand open up, the infinity of Sheila's life finally, thankfully released.

I hang up the phone and that's it—the shift is over. My ducks are all in a row and I can leave. Candace, Irving, Mr. Hampton, Sheila, and even Dorothy are no longer my patients. I am leaving, leaving, leaving. Another nurse, another good-hearted overworked soul in white will take over: night shift. And then tomorrow morning I'll be back.

But for now I do not think about tomorrow. Now is *now* and I am leaving. I prop my portable phone into one of the chargers at the nurses' station and am about to toss my papers in the shredder when I remember I may want them tomorrow. Throwing away my notes at the end of the shift always feels definitive, but it also makes me a little regretful. Legal requirements about patient confidentiality demand that my record of a day's work ends up as thin strips of cheap copy paper, confetti made from the records of four discrete people's lives.

Holding my notes, I head to the locker room and run into the owlish intern taking care of Mr. Hampton. He stops in the hall, head slightly bent, shoulders turned inward, exactly how he looked this morning. "He's doing OK with the Rituxan?" he asks. His voice is low and soft and he blinks at me behind his thick glasses.

"He's doing incredibly well," I tell him, explaining that Mr. Hampton stopped needing the oxygen, that he sat up on his own in bed, his confusion diminished, and enthusiastically took part in conversation. I smile and the intern, his slightly woebegone expression unchanged, focuses on my face as I keep talking. "I was so worried about him, and he did great."

"Well," he says, "If we could know the future our jobs would be a lot easier." He briefly makes full eye contact and I see again what I first liked about him this morning: underneath the tiredness, the working so hard just to stay afloat, there's a humaneness that impresses me. It surprises me to realize that I feel a bond with him and I felt it this morning, even though we had only a whisper of acquaintance informed by his workmanlike politeness and the scrupulousness that put him outside Mr. Hampton's room early in the morning.

I smile a trace of a smile at him and then scrunch together my eyebrows, thinking, *How can someone so young be so wise?*

As is so often the way in the hospital, we barely nod at each other and move on. Nurses and doctors—we come and go from our patients' lives and each other's with the anonymity of mail carriers, the efficient intimacy of the guy who reads the gas meter in the basement. That initial impression is what matters. Can I work with this person? Can I trust him?

In the locker room I take off my nurse shoes, put unused alcohol wipes and wrapped saline syringes back into my locker, toss in my notes from today with my pen clipped to the top, and pull out my tights for biking, along with my jacket and wraps. I'm making a reverse transformation from nurse back to ordinary person.

It's all women working tonight, so I dress quickly in the locker room instead of changing in the bathroom—it's one less step before I leave. I flatter myself that my black biking clothes peg me as a ninja, but I know I'm leaving the real action behind at the hospital. Besides, my bright yellow jacket completely ruins the ninja effect.

I run my ID card through the time clock and the computer asks me if I took a thirty-minute lunch break. I think we're supposed to hesitate before punching "no." It probably makes managers look bad if too many nurses say we didn't get lunch, whether we got our thirty minutes or not. I punch "no." The law's the law.

Slinging my bag over my shoulder, I jab the down button outside the elevator and then, unwilling to wait, take the stairs. I'm impatient, but the stairwell is also quiet. There are no speakers here so the overhead pages don't penetrate: no urgent calls for anesthesia, warnings about lost patients, or yet another fire drill will intrude. Down I go, down, down, down. The metal banister is cool under my hand and the cleats on my bike shoes make a gentle clicking noise on the stairs.

Halting briefly I glance out the window in the stairwell door and see a sign pointing right for the Medical ICU. *Mr. King,* I think. I slide my hand around the railing, stick my foot out to keep going down the stairs, then stop, turn and open the stairwell door and go through it, back into the hospital hallway.

I look again at the sign for the MICU and walk that way. ICU is a hard place for me since it's often the last stop for our sickest patients. We oncology nurses and the ICU RNs don't always get along so well, either. For some of us, the onc. patients are "ours" whether they're in the ICU or not and we can be critical of the care they receive there. ICU nurses feel we send them patients almost dead from treatment and expect miracles.

I push through the double doors, retrieve my name tag from my bag to show that I'm official, and try to look open and friendly. "We're all colleagues," I remind myself.

A nurse at the desk looks up questioningly at me and I

hold up my name tag. "I'm Theresa, here from medical oncology, wanting to see Frank King."

"He's, um, over there," she gestures, then returns to her charting.

"Who's his nurse?"

She looks up again, quickly, and reads down the whiteboard behind her. "Lemme see—it was Tim, but now it's . . . Eva."

"Cool. Thanks." She ignores me and continues working.

I walk by several rooms on my way to Mr. King's, seeing patients on ventilators, with multitudes of tubes and drips running in and out of them. The rooms are small and they beep and chirp from a variety of monitors and pumps.

I reach Mr. King's room, set down my bag, and look inside. There's a nurse with pale blond hair pulled back into a loose French braid standing by his bed.

"Are you Eva?"

She looks up, neutral. I show her my name tag. "Theresa, from upstairs," I point with my index finger. "I wanted to see how he's doing."

"He's awake," she says. "He just can't talk 'cause he's on the vent."

"He's awake? That's great." I step into the room and make eye contact, give a big smile. "Hi, Frank."

He blinks his eyes at me even though they're almost concealed by the breathing apparatus coming out of his mouth. He looks very frail, but at least blood's no longer dripping down his chin.

"Yeah, and his wife was in here earlier telling us this story about how she bought a dog for herself, but then the dog just fell in love with Frank and followed him everywhere and ignored her."

"Really?" I had never heard that story. I look right into his eyes. "Well, obviously, Frank, that dog knew quality."

Eva laughs and Frank's eyes crinkle together.

I take hold of his hand where it's lying on the sheet. "Listen, buddy—we all want what's best for you. You've been at this a long time." He blinks again.

"And everyone upstairs misses you." I squeeze his hand, but he gives no pressure back.

An X-ray tech comes to the door and I see his machine parked in the hallway outside. "Portable chest," he says. "You're gonna have to give me some room in here."

Eva looks up at me. She mouths, "Sorry," but I shake my head. "Is Opal here? His wife?"

"I think she went out to get something to eat." Eva shrugs, giving me a slight frown.

"This Xray was *STAT*," the technician says, walking into the room trailed by an assistant holding a flat sheet of film. "I need it *now*."

"Got it," I say. I squeeze Frank's hand one last time. "See you."

In the hallway I pull Eva aside. "What's the plan for him?"

She lowers her voice. "Family meeting tomorrow. His son can't get here until then and they want to make the decision about hospice together."

"Right. Well, thanks. He's a nice guy. We've taken care of him for a long time."

An alarm sounds in another room. "Eva, that's you," a voice calls out.

"Gotta go," she says, swirling around, her pale hair shining like light behind her.

I grab my bag from the floor and retrace my steps back to the stairwell. *It's over for Mr. King*, I think, and feel a lump forming in my throat. I shake my head, cough—it's not time to grieve; it's time to go home.

A few more flights down and at the first floor I open the heavy door slowly and walk out into an almost empty hallway. A couple of nurses are also leaving and a few visitors come and go. The cafeteria barely buzzes; they'll soon be closing up for the night. I can see why Opal would want to get food somewhere else.

The double glass doors whoosh open for me and, buttressed by a wall of indoor heated air, the evening's cold doesn't hit me until I take a few steps into it. After I've spent twelve hours in a hermetically sealed world, including a brief stop in the ICU, fresh air is enlivening. I breathe in, then feel the sting on my cheeks and pull my neck scarf up and over most of my face.

I unlock my bike, put on my helmet, snap the strap of my bag across my chest, and pull on my gloves. By the time I get home I'll be sweating, but right now I want to be comfortable, so I start out completely covered up. My bike lights are on and I zip straight out of the parking lot, happy that riding my bike makes parking free for me.

I push into traffic and the first real turn of the pedals is a release. The streets are dark and it's a weeknight, so there's very little traffic. My mind wanders to Dorothy. A few weeks before, she told me about her love of the Girl Scouts. It came up because she was trying to order a special Girl Scout hat and they kept messing up the order. I wonder how hard it would be to order one of those hats. How much might it cost? Could I surprise her with it? Pie in the sky—it'll never happen. For one thing, I can't afford to buy my patients gifts. But I'd like to get Dorothy the hat she wants if I could. Does that matter? My mother loves to say that the road to hell is paved with good intentions, but sometimes that's all we have in the hospital.

Pedal, breathe. I go slowly because I'm tired. I think about the owlish intern and his comment that knowing the future would make our jobs a lot easier.

Before I started this work I thought I would never be able to leave a patient at the hospital at the end of shift, never walk out when this trying chapter in someone's life story wasn't yet fully told. In nursing school, though, they teach us how to leave.

Clinical groups meet on the floor together at the start of shift and leave together at the end. We don't call the hospital after we've left to ask how so-and-so did. We give our all while we're there and then we go. This isn't indifference but practicality. Nurses are the hospital's mechanics, its sprockets and gears. The idea is, from one shift to another, a seamless blanket of nursing care is provided to every patient. For that model to work we have to make what happened that day—the good and the bad—as separate from ourselves as the uniforms we take off at shift's end.

And sometimes we don't know how a patient's story ends. People are "lost to follow up," move, get treatment elsewhere, never again come to the hospital because they're transferred to outpatient care. I often don't know what happens to patients I've laughed with, cried with, gone toe-to-toe with a doc for, or talked at length with family members about.

Pedal, breathe. I'm going uphill now over a short stretch of road paved with stones. Bumpity, bumpity. My hands shake on the handlebars but I go this way to avoid the smoothly paved but very steep road one block over.

Now Mr. Hampton's surprising, inexplicable recovery comes back to me. What if it continued? What if, after his dose of Rituxan is complete, he is completely healthy?

What if Mr. Hampton, his son Trace, and Trace's friend, Stephen, decide to begin a new life somewhere else? Where would that be? Spin the globe. Find some place warm, cheap. Could be an island, but the important thing is to be safe, hidden from disease and out of reach of modern medicine because he won't be needing it. It's my fantasy, creating for Mr. Hampton a new clean, well-lighted place.

The paving stones give way to asphalt and I turn right onto the last long climb to my house. The hill doesn't look that tough but it's a deceptively steady rise. This is where I start to sweat despite the winter's cold, give up on the idea of cadence, and just push slowly, breathing hard.

I let myself imagine Mr. Hampton and his family in the rain forest. They would build a house on a raised platform, fish for food, watch butterflies, listen to multi-colored birds squawk and scold, and laugh together. It will be warm but not too humid. If rain comes, it will be gentle. Time will stop.

And then I'm home. I go in through the basement so I can put away my bike. The dog comes down to greet me, sniffing and wagging her tail. Her dark coat shines in the basement's bare bulb lights. Upstairs I hear the clink of silverware, some news program on the radio. My husband will be finishing cooking dinner as he mulls current events or thinks about physics. The days I work, they wait on dinner so we all eat together.

I take off my helmet, gloves, unzip my Gore-tex. Home. I'm home again. The steps feel steeper than they did this morning, or maybe there are more of them. Finally at the top I reach up, pulling on the basement door, the old metal knob that's loose and rattly the way basement doorknobs should be.

Light hits me first and then more sounds. Not the bright fluorescent light of the hospital, but the soft incandescent lights of home. And not the beeps and rings and dings of the floor, but "Mom's home! Let's eat!" and the sound of my son practicing his violin.

"Do we need knives?" My daughters are setting the table.

"You made it," my husband says, looking up from the stove, as if I have come a long way just to get home for dinner. And maybe I have.

I turn off the radio and we eat: black beans, white rice, orange cheddar cheese, green broccoli, a glass of red wine. The meal is good and the wine gives me a start on feeling peaceful, but I'm not quite there yet.

The kids talk about school and I have no idea what they're saying. I'm thinking about Sheila. Sheila meeting with anesthesia. Sheila heading into the OR.

My husband plops a clear plastic container of mini peanut-butter cups on the table when we're done and I think of Dorothy's glass candy dish. I love that William Carlos Williams poem "So much depends / upon / a red wheel / barrow / glazed with rain / water / beside the white / chickens." A few of my fellow PhD students in graduate school derided that poem as a minimalist pretension to art written by a doctor pretending he was a poet. But those people never knew Dorothy or her candy dish, the pull it exerted on the staff, the way it told us something important about who she really was: a mother, generous, kind, with a determination to get what she wanted out of life.

After dinner I wash away memories in the shower, throw my dirty scrubs down the laundry chute, put on my pajamas. The shift is over. I settle into the threadbare couch in our family room and do the *New York Times* crossword puzzle in pen. Using ink is not about pride but aesthetics. Pencils scratch on newsprint and it's hard to see the traces of lead against the gray of the paper. The pen, in contrast, feels smooth and the strong capital letters I make stand out in the grid of squares.

The puzzle soothes me. I read a clue, "How knights roam," then fill in "ERRANTLY." Clever. Ordered. I may not be able to finish the whole thing, but that's only because some tricky logic, an extravagant pun, or the name of a European river or a small Oklahoma town eludes me. There is no fundamental deficiency in me that leads to failure to complete the grid, no lack of vigilance, or empathy, or efficiency, or ability to know that someone's belly hurts because part of her gut is torn, ripped open. No one will suffer if I never finish another crossword puzzle, if I Google all the answers and then lie about it, if I toss it into the recycling half done, without a backward glance.

I look up from the puzzle and my daughters are standing in front of me. Freshly showered themselves, with wet hair they refuse to brush, they call out to me, "Good night, Mom."

"Wait! Wait!" I say, startled out of my preoccupation with the puzzle and the day. "I have to hug you." It's almost exactly what I said to Sheila and I'm relieved that here with my own children there's so much less at stake.

One daughter extends her index finger and touches it to mine—the only version of a hug she allows me. The other, with only slight resistance, lets me slide an arm around her waist and squeeze. "Goodnight!" they chorus.

"Do you want me to come up and tuck you in?"

"No." Sometimes they say yes and I follow them up to their lair on the third floor of our house and then they tell me stories: the plot of a book one of them is reading, or what's up with Ultimate Frisbee, or this inexplicable thing Mr. So-and-So did in such-and-such class, or how funny Mrs. X is. Sometimes we even have girl talk about a lesson from health class or their surprisingly detailed middle-school sex education program.

Not tonight, though, and I don't fight it. Much as I hate to admit it I am pretty close to all used up.

My son, at fourteen an official teenager and biologically driven to stay up late, hauls his backpack into the family room. Then he roots around in it like a squirrel trying to find just the right nut from his store.

"Found it!" he says, extracting the piece of paper he needs.

"What is that?"

"Questions for U.S. History." I don't know if they're learning about the Revolutionary War, the Industrial Revolution, or the Underground Railroad.

"What are you studying now?"

"Stuff," he says, taking the piece of paper over to the computer and logging on to the course website.

"You know you need to sleep, right?"

"Uh-huh." He's reading online now.

"Well, OK." I walk over and give his shoulder a pat. "Good night. Don't stay up too late."

"Good night." he says, eagerly reading. Whatever he's studying, it has captured his imagination.

I go to brush my teeth and something about the ordinariness of that, the habit of it makes me think of Ray, Irving, and Candace, all pulled out of their regular lives and forced to confront the potentially deadly realities that accompany cancer.

"You going to bed?" It's my husband, come to check on me.

"Yuppers."

"You OK?"

I incline my head. "Why?"

"I don't know—you seem more out of it than you usually are after a shift."

I breathe in and let it out. "Today made no sense. My one patient I thought was fine wasn't at all, and my other patient, who I thought would maybe die from his treatment, did fantastically well."

"Aren't a lot of days like that? Isn't that why it's a hard job?"

"Are they?" Do I always live with this level of uncertainty and have never realized it? "I guess you're right." I tell him.

He places his index finger between my eyebrows and barely touches the worry wrinkle that I know has appeared. "Can you sleep?"

"I'll see," I tell him.

"'Cause I'm gonna stay up for a while . . ."

"That's fine. I'll try to sleep." He nods and leaves, turning out the light. I place my head on the pillow and then get up to look at the clock. It's 10:30 p.m. and I need to get up at 6:00 a.m. tomorrow. Sheila is God-knows-where in the hospital.

Sheila, Sheila, Sheila.

I rarely fall asleep easily after a shift, especially if I'm working the next one, but now quiescence comes, pushing at the edges of my mind. My breath deepens and I feel the calm of oblivion begin to cover me. I will do this all again tomorrow and then there will be another shift and another and another. To be in the eternal present of illness and unease, never knowing the future. It's where my patients live so I, ever hopeful, live there with them.

Knowing the Future

Peter didn't finish operating on Sheila until 2 a.m. and he told me her abdomen was full of stool. Shit. She had a belly full of shit. Peter and his team cut out the part of her colon that was dead and connected up the end of her living bowel to an outlet—a hole—in the wall of her abdomen. For the near future, and maybe for the rest of her life, she will defecate into a bag that attaches to the outside of her belly. It's called a colostomy and while it may sound distasteful or embarrassing, patients adapt. Even more important, they live.

I went down to the surgical ICU a couple times after Sheila's operation. Once I talked to her sister, the second time her nurse, but never to Sheila, who wasn't doing well. And then I got sick myself with a sinus infection and bronchitis. When I went back to work I was weak and had a hacking cough you could hear up and down the entire floor.

After a few weeks of dragging through my shifts I finally felt more or less like myself and sought out Sheila. She was on our inpatient surgery floor and I found time late one afternoon to stop by. But she was gone. The nurse said she'd left just a couple hours before—finally discharged after a month in the hospital.

I kept saying "What? She's gone?"

And Sheila's nurse kept saying, "It's really great you came down to see her. Really really great."

It didn't feel great but it didn't feel bad, either. In the end she did all right.

Beth's daughter made it home from Afghanistan OK, too. Apparently she took the world's longest shower once she arrived in the U.S. and then cut off her hair, so penetrating had been the Afghani dust. She visited Pittsburgh and went shopping with Beth, sat and talked outside while warding off fall's chill with their fire pit, got a chance to live without being under threat. "I never thought my daughter would end up a soldier," Beth told me one day at work, "but that's who she is."

Ray, Candace, and Irving all made it out of the hospital cancer-free. Their lives will continue to spool out as they each weave the fabric of their own unique existence.

Irving's story is the simplest. Whether by nature or as the result of his many troubles, Irving asked little of life and in that he was adequately answered. The group home kept him safe. The rocking chairs on the front porch were comfortable and the voices in his head weren't too intrusive or demanding. From him

I learned that sometimes when we strive less we end up with more of what we actually need.

Ray's brother's transplanted stem cells brought Ray back from the underworld. His journey was not as bad as it is for some though certainly rough enough. His skin didn't slough off, he wasn't cursed with voluminous black diarrhea, and despite a lifetime of enjoyably heavy drinking, his liver after treatment was none the worse for wear. He did succumb to infections, high fevers, breathing trouble, blood in his urine, but he came out whole.

His goal now, his mantra, is to stay out of the hospital unless he's critically ill, as defined by him. It's worked so far. He's returned to fighting fires. He plays in his band, loves his wife, is an involved father. The basics of life seem ordinary only if you've never faced losing them. His youth and health gave him only a slim advantage against his disease. He bet on his life and won.

And Candace. Unkind people might say that Candace sailed through her treatment because she was too mean for even cancer to hurt her. If only it were that easy. If only the right kind of personality could keep cells from duplicating out of control and clogging up veins and arteries and organs, forming tumors that grow their own blood supply and steal food from healthy tissue. If an optimist's cancer goes into remission we say that's the power of positive thinking. If it's someone like Candace we credit her survival to sheer cussedness.

There may be psychology involved, but it's never just that, and luck plays a big role, too. There's genetic luck always, sometimes at a level of biochemical processes that science does not yet understand. There's dumb luck, referring to when the cancer is detected, when treatment begins, and whether there's a match for transplant if a matched transplant (like Ray's) is what's needed. There's economic luck, too. Does the patient have good insurance that will pay for the best treatment available? Is she wealthy enough to cover a multitude of out-of-pocket costs without breaking the bank? And there's geographic luck as well. New Yorkers with cancer have more options than do South Dakotans or patients from Wyoming simply because they have a wider pool of nearby doctors and hospitals to choose from.

Candace may have saved her own life with her Clorox wipes and her obsessive hand washing. Evidence tells us that such attention to hygienic detail is relevant to what we euphemistically call "good outcomes," so it should not be described as pain-in-the-ass behavior but important work done by an "empowered patient," even though it's the kind of patient contribution that can make people who work in hospitals uncomfortable.

Despite all our good wishes Dorothy came back to the hospital several months later to die. Do we need the details? In the end she didn't even know herself much less anyone else. Her husband was there, taciturn, uncomfortably wedged into a too-small chair. Their daughter, whom I'd never met, but who had fielded many an annoyed and anguished phone call from Dorothy, was there, too. She looked like Dorothy with the same squat build except pale where Dorothy was dark. She talked to me about how Dorothy could be stubborn and demanding, and then her voice would start to shake and her eyes would fill with tears and she couldn't speak at all.

Dorothy didn't make it but her husband lived on, her daughter, too, and her granddaughter. Like it or not, this is the way life works; these are the terms we're all given, whether we accept them philosophically or resist with everything we've got.

I am sorry to report that after his treatment finished, Mr. Hampton did not go to the rain forest, he did not end his days listening to brightly colored birds and watching delicately winged butterflies. A few weeks after I was last his nurse I got to the hospital and learned he was checked in, too. I didn't see him—just his son, who had that irresistible smile, even though lines had crept onto his face. Around his eyes small creases gave away his stress and his look had an intensity that wasn't there before. Mr. Hampton's room was in the front part of the floor and my patients were in the very back.

"I thought you left," I called wishfully to Trace as I passed him in the hallway.

"We did, but then we came back," he told me, keeping his mouth straight and flat. And then I knew. His father had not had a miraculous recovery during his last hospital admission. Whatever happened to make him so much better while he slowly got Rituxan didn't last, which, sadly, was the more likely course of events for someone his age with his particular disease.

Trace was walking quickly, so I couldn't get more details then, but later on when I had the chance, I didn't ask Mr. Hampton's nurse how he was doing. I finished my shift in ignorance of his real fate and kept myself that way on purpose. In my mind he was living in a tropical paradise, eating freshly caught fish cooked just enough over an open flame. While that shift lasted I let myself believe that once I pushed Mr. Hampton's rock to the top of the health care hill it stayed there. Not true, I knew, but for those twelve hours I chose hope over hard reality.

Finally, a solid two years later at least, I ran into the owlish intern in my local coffee shop. I didn't remember his name and I'm pretty sure he didn't remember mine, and yet we knew each other right away. It turns out that we're neighbors.

He had become a fellow, not in oncology, and I debated with myself whether to speak up, to tell him about this book, and then I did. I told him he had said something so wise to me, something that shaped my thinking about the entire project: "If we could know the future our jobs would be a lot easier."

"That was probably something I said half asleep," he told me, not acting embarrassed or falsely modest, but being scrupulously honest, the way he had been so careful as an intern. He doesn't remember saying something that changed my life, but I do, and seeing him I felt the import of the entire shift again, for Mr. Hampton and for Sheila, for Candace, Dorothy, and Irving. I felt infinity in the palm of my hand and eternity over the next twelve very busy hours.

ACKNOWLEDGMENTS

Thanks to Jill Kneerim, agent, friend, and human being extraordinaire. I'm so glad to have you in my life. Amy Gash, who edited this book, made it so much better, in big ways and small. Working with Amy is like having an extra version of my own brain that always has the right answer.

The nurses, doctors, and patients on the Bone Marrow Transplant floor I write about here deserve much gratitude for being amazing colleagues and people. It was a privilege to work with all of you. Special thanks to people who read drafts of the book: Elizabeth Helsinger, Annie Im, Shannon Riskey, Josh Rubin, and my husband, Arthur Kosowsky. English professor, oncologist, oncology nurse practitioner, surgeon, and spouse. All of you were wonderful and helped tremendously.

Thanks also to Judith for mentioning Blake and providing thoughtful conversation as the book progressed, and to Julia, who always had my back. My editor at *The New York Times*, Clay Risen, wrote a book while I worked on this one and I really enjoyed discussing the process with him. Bob Miller, now at MacMillan, introduced me to Amy and helped get this project to Algonquin. Elisabeth Scharlatt and the marketing and publishing teams at Algonquin have been superlative throughout.

The nurses I worked with while writing this book charted its course and didn't mind (too much) when I worked less so I could write more: B. Byers, L. Marty, B. Mason, N. Palmquist, K. Smith, C. Spangler, and T. Reiser. Also L. Hartlein, the aide, and L. Harris, our amazing secretary who did seem able to be two places at once though I'm still not sure how she did it.

Friends, neighbors, and family members asked how the book was going, too many to list here, but know that your interest was always welcome, always supportive.

The character of Ray Mason is based on the life of Doug Weaver and his wife, Kalie Pierce. They both read the manuscript in draft and shared comments with me. Their only wish for the book was that I had named them "Sid and Nancy."

Families are often thanked last in acknowledgments and mine certainly did its part to bring this book to life. The kids are my inspiration for nursing and for success in writing. My husband never blinked when I decided to return to school to become a nurse. When I started writing about nursing he said full steam ahead. All of you are my everything. Many thanks.